I0790574

TOTAL FITNESS
For Women
U.S. Edition

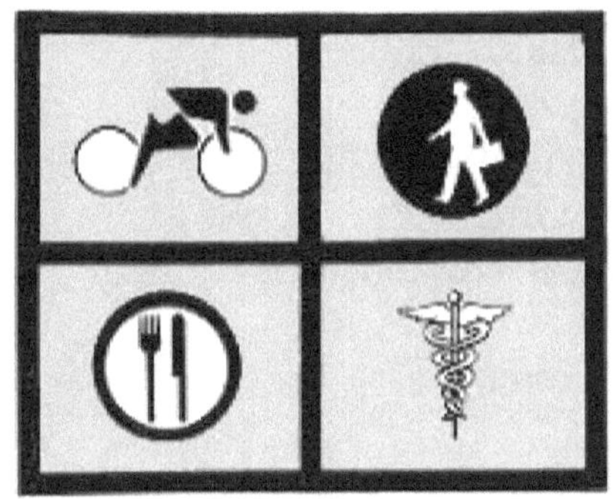

Vincent Antonetti, Ph.D.

NoPaperPress™

CONTENTS

WEIGHT MAINTENANCE

LIFE-LONG FITNESS

Disclaimer Statement

LIST OF TABLES

The person we call moderately active today, that is someone who walks an hour everyday and engages in some sport on the weekend, would have been considered sedentary a century ago! In many countries, the general lack of fitness of countless adults, who begin to show signs of old age – shortness of breath, obesity and clogged arteries – years earlier than their counterparts of just a few generations ago, is considered a national problem. The unfit person, who wants to call it a day two hours before quitting time and is obsessed with minor aches and pains, often lacks the vigor and physical toughness to cope with the long hours and high-stress that are part of the 21st century.

The fit person, on the other hand, typically has greater energy, tackles problems and projects head on, gets more done in less time, is better able to cope with stress, has a positive approach that is contagious, and does not get sick as often.

What's In This eBook

All aspects of fitness are covered in this text: exercise, weight control and, nutrition. The intent is to provide in a relatively complete form the facts needed for an in-depth understanding of all the components of a physical fitness program, and then to demonstrate how this information can be used to plan and implement a successful personal fitness program.

Medical personnel, health education specialists, personal fitness trainers, and corporate fitness directors should find the data in this edition useful in devising or supervising physical fitness programs. Whether this book is used as a professional reference, or as a personal fitness guide, the aim is to provide the facts and data needed to achieve and maintain a healthful physical fitness level.

Health Risks & Counter Measures

Four of the leading causes of death in the United States are heart disease, cancer, stroke and diabetes. That's the bad news. The good news is that research indicates that people who exercise regularly, who eat the right foods and who maintain a normal weight, i.e., who are physically fit, can reduce their risk of heart attack, stroke and diabetes, and also gain some protection against certain forms of cancer. Although it is not possible completely stop these diseases, enough is known to prevent many - if not most - premature incidents. For every health risk there is a counteracting step you can take.

No one set of rules will guarantee health or fitness. Age, gender, and physical condition are all factors in determining the specific program that is best for you. We can delineate, however, seven guidelines for a total fitness program:

- Have periodic medical checkups

- Do not smoke
- Practice good nutrition habits
- Exercise regularly
- Maintain a proper weight level
- Learn to relax
- Drink alcoholic in moderation

The Benefits of Being Fit

Although our primary aim is to reduce the risk of cardiovascular illness, stroke, cancer and diabetes, physical fitness is much more than not being sick or merely being well. It is a positive quality. Ideally, it is the ability to withstand stress, and to persevere under circumstances where an unfit person would quit. While the results will differ from individual to individual, most often **being fit will result in a longer life expectancy, less illness, a healthful appearance, the ability to work (and play) with vigor and an energy reserve for emergencies.**

Everyone knows regular exercise improves your strength and flexibility and can help you lose weight. But did you know that regular exercise promotes the loss of fat rather than muscle and other nonfat tissue? Research also shows that people who include regular exercise as part of their weight-loss program are more likely to keep off the weight they have lost than people who only changed their diet.

Not so evident, but perhaps even more important, are the beneficial changes in the functioning of the heart, lungs and circulatory system. Physical activity lowers your risk of developing heart disease and helps control blood pressure and diabetes. The heart is a pump made of muscle. Just as exercise strengthens the other muscles in your body, it also strengthens your heart. With exercise your heart beat becomes stronger and steadier, breathing becomes deeper, and circulation improves. In more specific terms, a well-designed total fitness program – encompassing exercise, nutrition and weight control – will:

- Reduce your risk of disease
- Lower your blood pressure
- Result in a stronger & more efficient heart
- Keep your arteries supple and young
- Speed up your basal metabolism
- Help you lose weight
- Convert fat to muscle
- Build larger more powerful muscles
- Strengthen your bones

Longevity: Being fit can't quite turn back the clock but it can make you look and feel younger than your chronological age – and you will probably live longer too. There are a number of scientific studies that conclude that regular exercise improves the quality of life in old age and actually prolongs life by more than two years when compared to sedentary individuals.

In fact, according to the Harvard School of Public Health, your life expectancy increases about two hours for every hour of regular exercise. So we should add the following to our list of benefits of being fit:
- You will probably live longer
- You will look & feel younger than your actual age

Knowledge is Power

Certainly, the desire to be fit and the discipline to start and stay on a fitness program are crucial. But along with desire and discipline, it is our belief that **only an in-depth understanding of exercise, nutrition and weight control will lead to long-term success**. As is true with many important and complex subjects, to achieve you need more than rules – you need a solid understanding.

Stated or not, everyone has goals in mind when they embark on a physical fitness program. It could be reducing the risk of illness, losing weight, improving your appearance, or becoming stronger. Before you begin your program, however, you should know where you stand, i.e., your current fitness level. Assessing your current level in areas such as aerobic (cardio) capacity, strength, flexibility, percent body-fat, and even how appropriate your nutritional practices are, will help you establish what you should emphasize in your physical fitness program and help you set goals.

Medical Assessment

Everyone should have a medical assessment, or exam, before starting a physical fitness program. The medical checkup may be as simple as a visit to a physician who is familiar with your medical history, or it may be a thorough physical exam. In all cases the physician conducting the medical exam should be made aware of and should approve the specific physical fitness program you're planning. In addition, if you have or suspect you have cardiovascular disease or other health problems, if you are obese, if you have been totally inactive, or if you are 40 or older, before embarking on a physical fitness program you should have a stress test supervised by a physician. Specific age-dependent guidelines are as follows:

Ages 20-29: For most young people in this age group a medical checkup will probably be a rather quick, basic medical exam.

Ages 30-39: The medical exam is somewhat more extensive for this age group and should include a resting EKG.

<u>**Ages 40-59**</u>: Those in this age category should proceed with still more care by having an exercising or stress-type EKG as part of their medical exam.

<u>**Ages 60 +:**</u> The medical checkup for people in this category is basically the same as for the 40-59 year olds.

Some gyms, health clubs and fitness centers also offer a complete fitness evaluation where your aerobic capacity, strength, flexibility and body-fat percentage are determined before you sign on to a program. Besides being a good indicator of what sort of shape you are in, these tests give you a baseline you can use to judge your progress after some time on a fitness program. Alternatively, you can also get a good indication of your overall condition by taking some body measurements and performing a few simple tests as outlined in the following pages.

Cardio Self Assessment

A good measure of aerobic capacity, or cardio-respiratory fitness, is the volume of oxygen per minute per kilogram of body weight (called VO_{2max}) a person can process during hard exercise. Higher values of VO_{2max} indicate better aerobic fitness. For example, a 25 year-old man in excellent physical condition can process about 50 milliliters of oxygen per minute per kilogram of body weight; compared to less than 20 mL/min/kg for a 70 year-old woman in poor condition.

One of the best self assessment tests for VO_{2max} is the <u>Rockport Walking Test</u>. This is a field test, not a laboratory test, and consists of walking one mile as rapidly as you can. At the end of the test you record your pulse and the time required to complete the walk. Then convert the time to completion and your pulse into VO_{2max} using the formulae (on the next page). Lastly, you enter the Table 1 with your calculated VO_{2max} and determine your cardio-respiratory fitness level.

There is some risk if you take the Rockport Fitness Walking Test without prior conditioning. That is why I recommend the following precautions.

1) Be sure to have a medical exam before taking the walking test.

2) If you are over 30 years old, postpone the walking test until you have been exercising regularly for at least one month.

3) You must be able to walk comfortably at least two miles before you take the walking test.

4) When you take the test, if you feel exhausted, experience shortness of breath, become dizzy or light headed, or nauseous, stop the test. Do not attempt a retest until you have seen a physician and exercised regularly for at least another three months, when your fitness level should have improved.

The One-Mile Walking Test: If available, walk on a school track or a measured and marked flat trail with a smooth surface. (An older standard track is one-quarter mile, so walk four laps on the inside lane for the one-mile test.) You also can use a treadmill rather than a track. Although not as accurate, if need be you can walk a street course you have driven and measured.

Before you start the test, warm up for several minutes with easy walking and stretching. Rest for about one minute. Then start the test. Walk as briskly as possible for one mile, but remember you'll probably walk at least 12 minutes, so don't start too fast. Pick up the pace on the last lap if you still feel strong. When you finish the test, it's important to immediately measure your pulse. (See page 35 for recommended pulse measurement techniques.) At the conclusion of the test, you should feel slightly winded, but you should not be gasping for air. Your goal is to end the test feeling tired but not exhausted. Remember to cool down by continuing to walk slowly for a few minutes.

Table 1: VO2max versus Fitness Level

Age	Cardio-Respiratory Fitness Level			
	Poor	**Fair**	**Good**	**Excellent**
20-29	23.6-28.9	29.0-32.9	33.0-36.9	37.0-41.0
30-39	22.8-26.9	27.0-31.4	31.5-35.6	35.7-40.0
40-49	21.0-24.4	24.5-28.9	29.0-32.8	32.9-36.9
50-59	20.2-22.7	22.8-26.9	27.0-31.4	31.5-35.7
60+	17.5-20.1	20.2-24.4	24.5-30.2	30.3-31.4

Calculating VO_{2max}: The following is undoubtedly the most difficult computation in this book, because VO_{2max} is a function of so many variables: gender, weight, age, heart rate and time to complete the one-mile test walk. Although the formulae are relatively complex, we have tried to simplify the calculation as much as possible. The formula for women is:

$VO_{2max} = 133 - W - H - A - T$, where

    $W = 0.077 \times$ Weight

    $A = 0.39 \times$ Age

    $H = 0.157 \times$ Heart rate

    $T = 3.26 \times$ Time for mile

<u>**Example**</u>: Determine VO_{2max} and the fitness level of a 29 year-old woman who weighs 150 pounds. She finished the one-mile walking test in 14 minutes and 30 seconds (which is 14.5 minutes) with a heart rate of 145 beats per minute. The first step is to determine values for W, H, A and T.

W = 0.077 × Weight = 0.077 × 150 lbs = 11.6

H = 0.157 × Heart rate = 0.157 × 145 = 22.8

A = 0.39 × Age = 0.39 × 29 years = 11.3

T = 3.26 × Time = 3.26 × 14.5 minutes = 50.5

Then calculate VO_{2max} = 133 – W – H – A – T

VO_{2max} = 133 – 11.6 – 22.8 – 11.3 – 50.5 = 36.8

Finally, enter Table1 and find that a 29 year-old woman with VO_{2max} = 36.8, her fitness level is good – actually very good bordering on excellent.

Strength Assessment

Rather than a strength-assessment that consists of one repetition with a maximum load, I prefer the much safer anaerobic muscular strength measuring technique, where you assess your strength by the number of repetitions you can perform with a sub-maximal load. Moreover, in the tests that follow you will use your own body weight to determine how strong you are. The standard tests are: the push-up test, the sit-up test, and the squat test. Because the sit-up test can aggravate existing lower back problems, I only recommend the push-up and squat tests. The objective in both tests is to see how many push-up and squat repetitions you can perform without stopping.

<u>**Push-up Test**</u>: For the test, women should employ the familiar half push-up, supporting their weight with their arms and knees. Use Table 2 to assess your performance.

Table 2: Pushup Performance

Age	Push-up Performance		
	Below Average	Average	Above Average
20-29	0 - 16	17 - 33	34 - 50
30-39	0 - 11	12 - 24	25 - 37
40-49	0 - 7	8 - 19	20 - 29
50-59	0 - 5	6 - 14	15 - 23
60+	0 - 2	3 - 5	6 - 8

<u>**Squat Test**</u>: Stand about 12 inches in front of a chair. Place your feet about shoulder width apart and extend your arms parallel to the floor to your front. Bend your knees and slowly lower your body until your butt just touches the seat of the chair. (But don't sit on the chair.) Then slowly return to the standing position. Repeat as often as you can without stopping. Use Table 3 to assess your performance.

Age	Squat Test Performance		
	Below Average	Average	Above Average
20-29	17 - 19	21 - 23	24 - 26
30-39	15 - 17	18 - 20	21 - 23
40-49	12 - 14	15 - 17	18 - 20
50-59	9 - 11	12 - 14	15 - 17
60+	6 - 8	9 - 11	12 - 14

Table 3 Squat-Test Performance

Flexibility Assessment

Sit & Reach Test: This is a standard test to determine hip and trunk flexibility and is often used as a measure of overall flexibility. Remember to warm up with a few gentle stretches before you start the test. To conduct the test, tape a yardstick to the floor at the 15-inch mark. Remove your shoes and sit on the floor, with your legs forward and fully extended, so that the yardstick is between and almost parallel to your extended legs. (The yardstick's zero mark should be closest to you). Locate your heels at the 15-inch mark and move your feet about 10 inches apart. Place one hand over the other and slowly stretch forward (without jerking or bouncing), and extend the tips of your fingers as far as possible along the yardstick. Repeat three times. Your score is the furthest or highest number you are able to reach. Use Table 4 to assess your flexibility.

Age	Sit & Reach Test Performance		
	Below Average	Average	Above Average
20-29	14.5 - 17.4	17.5 - 20.5	20.6 - 23.5
30-39	13.5 - 16.4	16.5 - 19.5	19.6 - 22.5
40-49	10.0 - 14.4	14.5 - 19.0	19.1 - 22.0
50-59	10.0 - 14.4	14.5 - 17.5	17.6 - 20.5
60+	10.0 - 13.9	14.0 - 17.0	17.1 - 20.0

Table 4 Sit & Reach Test

Body-Weight Assessment

In recent years, many health-care practitioners rely on Body Mass Index, or BMI, to determine if a person is overweight. The BMI takes into account both a person's weight and height and is calculated by dividing a person's weight in kilograms by the square of their height (in meters). Table 5 provides a convenient determination of BMI for U.S. readers. This table is not applicable to competitive athletes, body builders and the chronically ill.

Weight (lbs.)	- Height -									
	60"	62"	64"	66"	68"	70"	72"	74"	76"	78"
100	19.6	18.3								
110	21.5	20.1	18.9	17.8						
120	23.5	22.0	20.6	19.4	18.3					
140	27.4	25.6	24.0	22.6	21.3	20.1	19.0			
160	31.3	29.3	27.5	25.8	24.3	23.0	21.7	20.6	19.5	
180	35.2	33.0	30.9	29.0	27.4	25.8	24.4	23.1	21.9	20.8
200	39.1	36.6	34.3	32.3	30.4	28.7	27.1	25.7	24.3	23.1
220	43.0	40.3	37.8	35.5	33.4	31.3	29.8	28.2	26.8	25.4
240	46.9	43.9	41.2	38.7	36.5	34.4	32.6	30.8	29.2	27.8
260	50.8	47.6	44.7	42.0	39.5	37.3	35.3	33.4	31.6	30.1
280		51.3	48.1	45.2	42.6	40.2	38.0	35.9	34.1	32.4
300			51.5	48.5	45.6	43.0	40.7	38.6	36.5	34.7
400							54.3	51.4	48.7	46.3

Table 5 Body Mass Index (BMI)

BMI	Weight Profile
18.5 or less	Underweight
18.6 to 24.9	Normal
25.0 to 29.9	Overweight
30.0 to 39.9	Obese
40 or more	Extremely Obese

Table 6 Weight Profile vs. BMI

The rationale behind the BMI is based on epidemiological data that show an increase in mortality when the BMI is above 25, although the increase in mortality tends to be moderate until a BMI of 30 is reached. Table 6 shows how a person's body-weight is categorized as a function of their BMI.

BMI-Based Weight vs. Height

A better way to use BMI is the **New** BMI-Based Weight vs. Height Chart shown in Table 7, where the underweight category corresponds to BMI = 18.5 or less, normal weight is for BMI = 18.6 to 24.9, overweight is for BMI

= 25.0 to 29.9, obese is for BMI = 30.0 to 39.9 and extremely obese is for BMI = 40 or more.

Table 7 BMI-Based Weight vs. Height

Height	Normal	Overweight	Obese
4' 10"	90 – 119	120 – 142	143 – 191
4' 11"	93 – 123	124 – 148	149 – 197
5' 0"	96 – 127	128 – 152	153 – 204
5' 1"	99 – 131	132 – 158	159 – 211
5' 2"	102 – 135	136 – 163	164 – 218
5' 3"	105 – 140	141 – 169	170 – 225
5' 4"	109 – 144	145 – 173	174 – 232
5' 5"	112 – 149	150 – 180	181 – 239
5' 6"	116 – 154	155 – 185	186 – 247
5' 7"	119 – 159	160 – 191	192 – 254
5' 8"	123 – 163	164 – 196	197 – 262
5' 9"	126 – 168	169 – 202	203–270
5' 10"	130 – 173	174 – 206	207 – 278
5' 11"	134 – 178	179 – 214	215 – 286
6' 0"	137 – 183	184 – 220	221 – 294
6' 1"	141 – 188	189 – 227	228 – 302
6' 2"	145 – 194	195 – 232	233 – 310
6' 3"	149 – 199	200 – 239	240 – 319
6' 4"	152 – 205	206 - 246	247 - 328
6' 5"	157 - 210	211 - 252	253 – 337
6' 6"	161 - 216	217 - 259	260 - 346

Example: Determine BMI of a 5' 6" woman who weighs 160 pounds.
First use Table 5. Scan the far left of the table and locate her weight of 160 pounds. From this number run your finger horizontally (to the right) until it intersects the vertical column headed by her 5' 6" height. The number at the intersection is her BMI = 25.8. According to Table 6 she is slightly overweight.

<u>**Example**</u>: Determine the normal (healthy) weight range for a woman who is 5' 6" tall.

From Table 7, find that at 5' 6" she must weigh between 116 and 154 pounds for her weight to be in the "normal" range, that is for her BMI to be between 18.6 and 24.9. I think you will agree that the new BMI-Based Weight vs. Height chart (Table 7) is more useful than the BMI table (Table 5).

<u>**Waist-to-Hip Ratio**</u>: Another important weight-profile parameter is your waist-to-hip ratio. Health risks for heart attack and stroke increase considerably for men with a ratio above 1.0 and for women with a ratio above 0.8. To calculate your ratio, measure your waist size (at its narrowest circumference) and divide it by your hip size (at the widest section).

Are You Eating Sensibly?

To broadly assess how appropriate your current nutritional practices are please complete the following questionnaire. (You may need pencil and paper to keep your score.)

a) Number of vegetable servings eaten per day?
   None (1 point), 1 serving (2 points), 2 to 4 (3 points), 5 or more (4 points)

b) How many fruit servings do you eat in a day?
   None (1 point), 1 serving (2 points), 2 to 4 (3 points), 5 or more (4 points)

c) Cereal & whole-grain bread servings in a day?
   None (1 pt), 1 serving (2 pts), 2 to 4 (3 pts), 5 or more (4 pts)

d) How many times per week do you eat a fish or poultry?
   Never (1 pt), 1 time (2 pts), 2 to 3 (3 pts), 4 or more (4 pts)

e) How do you prepare and eat poultry?
   Fry dark meat with skin & gravy (1 pt)
   Bake or broil dark meat with skin & gravy (2 pts)
   Bake or broil dark meat without skin (3 pts)
   Bake or broil white meat without skin (4 pts)

f) How many times per week do you eat beans, lentils, peas?
   Never (1 pt), 1 time (2 pts), 2 to 3 (3 pts), 4 or more (4 pts)

g) How often per week do you eat burgers, salami, frankfurter, bacon, etc?
   7 or more (1 pt), 4 to 6 (2 pts), 2 to 3 (3 pts), Rarely (4 pts)

h) When you consume milk, yogurt, ice cream, etc, you most often select:
   Only whole-fat dairy product (1 pt)
   Whole milk, but low-fat yogurt & ice cream (2 pts)
   Low-fat (1 or 2% fat) (3 pts)
   Skim or non-fat products (4 pts)

i) If ordering potatoes in a restaurant would you choose:
   French fried or hash brown (1 pt)

Baked or boiled with butter and/or sour cream (2 pts)
Boiled without butter or sour cream (3 pts)
Baked without butter or sour cream (4 pts)

j) How many times per week do you eat fast-food?
5 or more (1 pt)
3 or 4 times (2 pts)
1 or 2 (3 pts)
Rarely (4 pts)

k) Do you add salt to your food?
At every meal (1 pt)l
Once per day (2 pts)
2 or 3 times per week (3 pts)
Rarely (4 pts)

l) How often do you eat sweets (cookies, candy bar, etc)?
More than one sweet per day (1 pt)
About one per day (2 pts)
2 to 4 sweets per week (3 pts)
Rarely (4 pts)

m) Do you take any vitamin or mineral supplements?
None (1 pt)
Take herbal supplements (2 pts)
Take individual vitamins (like C, E, etc) (3 pts)
Take multi-vitamin & mineral supplement (4 pts)

n) If you want to lose weight, how do you proceed?
Go on a crash die (1 pt)
Stop eating carbs (2 pts)
Cut back on carbs & increase exercise (3 pts)
Reduce caloric intake & increase exercise (4 pts)

This completes our brief nutrition practices assessment. Add up your score and see how you compare to the following standards.
Excellent = 49 to 56 points
Good = 41 to 48
Fair = 32 to 40
Poor = 23 to 31
Very Poor = 14 to 22

Time to Set Goals

To this point, we defined the problem; then we outlined a "fitness prescription," and next we briefly set forth techniques you can use to assess your aerobic capacity, your strength, your flexibility, your body weight, and your nutritional practices, i.e., your current total fitness level.

Now it's time to review your fitness-self-assessment test results and set some broad personal fitness goals, such as losing weight and improving your aerobic capacity. You're not quite ready to construct a total program. That will have to wait until you read the exercise, nutrition and weight control chapters. These topics are somewhat complex and are treated in depth in the pages that follow.

EXERCISE FUNDAMENTALS

Many of us exist largely through mental efforts - by our wits and skill. All the advances of modern technology – from washing machines to automobiles to computers – have made life easier, or at least physically much less demanding. For most people, the common tasks of living and working no longer provide enough exercise to develop and maintain cardiovascular and respiratory fitness and good muscle tone. With any luck we can go for weeks without working up a good sweat or drawing a deep breath! Our bodies, however, are virtually identical to that of primitive humans who survived through physical efforts – by strength and stamina.

In fact, the bodies we inherited are just not built to be immobile and passive. The sad fact, however, is that after years of education and information programs by government agencies and medical associations relatively few Americans engage in regular planned exercise – despite the reality that we need to be active to keep our systems working efficiently and to rid ourselves of emotional tension. There are two ways to become more physically active: 1) Increase the physical activity in your daily life; and 2) Start on a regular exercise program. Better still would be a combination of both.

Be More Active Every Day

Before we address exercise programs, here are some ways you can increase physical activity in your daily routine:

Change your attitude toward the occasional "bothersome" physical tasks that you encounter in daily living. Consider anytime you have to lift, bend, reach, walk, as an opportunity to burn additional calories and as an extension of your formal workout.

Look for opportunities to walk, such as walking up stairs (two at a time if you can) rather than using an elevator, walking to a local store rather than driving, walking the course if you play golf, and mowing your lawn. At work stand up and stretch two or three times a day, read standing up, etc.

Engage in leisure activities such as dancing, bowling and gardening more often. They can be enjoyable and provide added exercise.

Each of these daily activities taken alone may not seem like much, but done every day for many years they can add up to a substantial number of extra calories burned.

Calories Burned

Table 8 shows the number of calories burned per hour for various activities. Although the data in the table are from reliable sources, you may find that some of the values are slightly different than those in other books. There are several reasons for this. First, the intensity of the activity being measured may actually vary (for instance handball can be played at many different levels – with a different number of calories burned at each level). Then the calories burned by same-weight individuals engaged in the same activity does vary somewhat; and finally measurement techniques and data collection accuracy vary slightly from laboratory to laboratory. The best one can do, therefore, is arrive at an average from the available data, which often requires judgment and compromise. More important, notice that the calories expended for a given activity depends on your weight. Good news: **For any activity, the more you weigh the more calories you burn!**

<u>**Example**</u>: Determine the number of calories burned by a 187-pound woman (or man) who walks seven miles in two hours.

First calculate the person's walking speed = 7 miles / 2 hours = 3.5 mph. Because 187 lbs is not listed in Table 8, we use the neighboring weight of 180 lbs. Then from Table 8 we find that walking at 3.5 mph a 180-pound person burns 357 Calories per hour.

Thus, in two hours a 180-pound person would burn 2 x 357 = 714 Calories.

But from this we must subtract the number of calories a 180-pound person would have used anyway if, instead of walking, he or she just sat for the two hours. From Table 8 this amounts to 105 Calories per hour, or 210 Calories in two hours.

Then the net energy a 180-pound person would expend walking (over and above just sitting) totals 714 – 210 = 504 Calories.

However, the woman in this example weighs 187 pounds and would expend proportionately more calories than a 180-pound person, or 504 x 187 / 180 = <u>524 Calories</u>

Activity	Weight (lbs.)								
	120	140	160	180	200	220	240	260	280
Aerobics (dance)	491	573	655	736	818	900	982	1064	1145
Basketball	382	445	509	573	636	700	764	827	891
Bicycle (13 mph)	435	508	580	653	725	798	870	943	1015
Calisthenics	341	398	455	511	568	625	682	739	795
Dancing	250	292	333	375	417	458	500	542	583
Golf (pull cart)	270	315	360	405	450	495	540	585	630
Golf (riding cart)	190	222	253	285	317	348	380	412	443
Handball	365	426	487	548	609	670	731	792	853
Hiking	320	373	427	480	533	587	640	693	747
Hockey	430	502	573	645	717	788	860	932	1003
Horseback riding	215	251	287	323	358	394	430	466	502
Jog (8 min mile)	680	793	907	1020	1133	1247	1360	1473	1587
Mowing lawn	299	349	399	449	499	549	599	649	699
Raking leaves	328	383	438	493	547	602	657	711	766
Rowing	380	443	507	570	633	697	760	823	887
Sitting	70	82	93	105	117	128	140	152	163
Skating	380	443	507	570	633	697	760	823	887
Skiing +country	435	508	580	653	725	798	870	943	1015
Skiing (downhill)	330	385	440	495	550	605	660	715	770
Skipping rope	457	533	609	686	762	838	914	990	106
Soccer	410	479	547	615	684	752	820	889	957
Softball	270	315	360	405	450	495	540	585	630
Spinning	382	445	509	573	636	700	764	827	891
Squash	365	426	487	548	609	670	731	792	853
Swimming laps	440	513	587	660	733	807	880	953	1027
Tennis (singles)	320	373	427	480	533	587	640	693	747
Tennis (doubles)	243	283	324	364	405	445	485	526	566
Walk (3mph)	194	227	259	291	324	356	388	421	453
Walk (3.5 mph)	238	277	317	357	396	436	476	515	555
Walk (4 mph)	302	353	403	453	504	554	604	655	705

Table 8: Calories Burned for Various Activities

Types of Exercise

Simply stated there are **three basic types of exercise: aerobic, stretching, and strengthening**.

<u>**Aerobic exercises**</u> (also called "cardio") condition your cardiovascular system. Aerobic exercises, such as jogging, swimming, cycling, brisk walking, skipping rope, jogging in place, and many others, are typically deep breathing and continuous, with rhythmic and repetitive contractions of your large muscle groups. Most aerobic exercises have one thing in common: they make you work hard and require you to process a great deal of oxygen.

Aerobic is a word derived from the Greek, meaning "with oxygen." Aerobic activities require oxygen for the production of energy. The main goal of an aerobic exercise program is to increase the rate which your body can process oxygen, i.e., increase VO_{2max}. A well-conditioned person with efficient lungs and a strong heart can pump large volumes of blood, can breathe large volumes of air, and via the blood circulatory system effectively transport the oxygen in the air they breathe to all parts of their body.

During aerobic exercise, the large muscles of the body continuously flood the heart with a great deal of blood; the heart beats faster; blood flow rate increases; and the lungs transport large quantities of oxygen to the blood. Regular exercise of this type "trains" the heart to pump more blood with less effort. Aerobic exercise improves the circulatory system by developing more elastic arteries and by creating peripheral or extra blood paths to the heart; and aerobic exercise strengthens the muscles of respiration increasing the volume of oxygen that can be processed within a given time. Done regularly, aerobic exercises improve stamina and endurance, and most importantly promote what should be your central exercise goal - cardiovascular fitness. For if your cardiovascular system is not in shape, you're not in shape - no matter how many push-ups or crunches you can do! In net, aerobic exercises develop a powerful heart, an effective circulatory system and efficient lungs.

Aerobic exercises can be further subdivided according to how strenuous they are and how well they condition the heart and lungs. (Note, there are exercises other than those shown that could be included in the groupings that follow.)

<u>**Group A:**</u> Basketball, Cross-country skiing, Dancing (aerobic), Hiking in rugged terrain, Ice Hockey, Jogging, Jogging in place, Rowing, Skipping rope, Stair climbing, and Stationary cycling.

<u>**Group B:**</u> Bicycling Field Hockey, Calisthenics, Handball, Racquetball, Skiing (downhill), Soccer, Squash, Tennis (singles), Volleyball, and Walking (briskly).

<u>**Group C:**</u> Badminton, Baseball, Bowling, Croquet, Dancing, Gardening, Golf (carrying or pulling clubs), Horseback riding, Housework, Ping-pong, Shuffleboard, Softball, Tennis (doubles) and Walking (moderate to leisurely).

The vigorous exercises in Group A are intended for those already in good condition who want to further strengthen their heart and lungs and improve their aerobic capacity. The moderate exercises in Group B are not as demanding as those in Group A, but they are nevertheless good choices and can condition your heart and lungs. The exercises in Group C are actually not aerobic because they are either low intensity or not continuous, or both, but they still can be beneficial in that they improve muscle tone and coordination, relieve tension and burn some calories. (Note that some exercises in one group if done vigorously could easily be as demanding as those in the next higher grouping. For example, a very intense game of squash could move it from the Group B to the Group A category.)

As a final point, please note that the exercise portion of *Total Fitness for Women* is aimed at the beginner who wants to improve his or her fitness level and general health, and someone who has already attained some degree of fitness but wants to learn more and go on to the next level. It is not intended for individuals who want to be highly-conditioned athletes and so topics such as interval, tempo and uphill training methods are not covered. (On the other hand, people at all fitness levels will find the information in the "Nutrition Basics" and "Weight Control" sections extremely valuable.)

<u>**Stretching-type exercises**</u> such as yoga, tai chi, Pilates and to a lesser extent calisthenics can improve your flexibility – and some of the exercises can make you somewhat stronger.

As you age you inevitably start to loose flexibility. Your gait becomes stiffer; you can't stand quite as upright as you used to; it becomes tougher to bend over; and you have difficulty turning your neck. Regardless of your age, however, stretching can make you more flexible, less injury prone, and can reduce the pain and discomfort associated with tight muscles and shortened tendons. Realize, however, that stretching exercises do not condition your heart and lungs. Stretching exercises are fine as long as they are performed in addition to rather than in place of an aerobic exercise.

Most experts do recommend stretching before and after aerobic and strength routines. However, never stretch cold muscles and always do some form of warm up prior to stretching. Stretch slowly and hold gently. You should stretch to the point of feeling a mild pull, but you should never feel pain. And when you stretch – do not bounce.

<u>**Muscle building** and **strengthening exercises,**</u> e.g., weight lifting, use of the machines found in fitness centers and isometrics.

Once more, as you age you loose muscle mass, your bone density decreases and you lose strength. Exercises like weight lifting strengthen your muscles, bones and joints. Strengthening exercises also reduce your risk of developing osteoporosis, a severe bone-loss disease, which can lead to easily fractured bones and all the complications that often follow. Strong muscles not only allow you to lift a sleepy four-year old out of a car without difficulty and lug groceries up to a second floor apartment, but as with increased flexibility, strong muscles also make you less injury prone. **Strengthening exercises are beneficial and should be a part of your fitness routine, but again they should be performed in addition to an aerobic exercise** because alone they cannot condition your heart and lungs.

Select the Right Exercise

Selecting the right fitness exercise is the key to a successful conditioning program. You should try to pick an activity (or activities) you will enjoy. Factors to consider in choosing your activity are: your medical condition, your age, your fitness level, your exercise goals, your daily and overall schedule, exercise outdoors or indoors, exercise alone or with others, and how much money you are prepared to spend. You may decide to concentrate on one activity such as squash, or you may choose to walk briskly some days and lift weights on other days. Incidentally, three to five days of a vigorous aerobic exercise plus two days of either strength or flexibility exercises per week is a good combination. Whatever you settle on make sure it is an activity (or activities) that can be done regularly and that you enjoy.

Your Medical Condition: If you have a medical condition such as a heart problem, diabetes, osteoporosis, etcetera, or if you are a female who is pregnant or breast-feeding, you should proceed with caution, and be sure to talk to your doctor before you start any exercise activity. See the page 10 for the section on **Medical Assessment** and for age-related recommendations.

Your Fitness Level: If you have been inactive for some time, rather than starting with one of the more strenuous exercises, **beginners of all ages should initially confine themselves to walking** until they can easily walk two miles at a brisk pace. When you reach this stage more strenuous exercises can be attempted if desired. Furthermore, some sports medicine physicians contend that **if you are badly overweight you should limit your exercise to walking** until you have lost weight to the point where you are less than 25 percent overweight.

Your Exercise Goals: If you want to strengthen your heart and lungs, improve your aerobic capacity and burn a lot of calories select an aerobic activity from Group A or B. If you want to improve your flexibility select a stretching type exercise. And if you want to become physically stronger choose one of the strength-building exercises.

Your Schedule: Only you know what the demands on your time from work, family and your social life are. What is the best time of day for you? Which days of the week best fit your schedule? Of course, you must be open to rearranging your priorities to fit exercise into your daily life.

Outdoors or Indoors: If you decide to exercise outdoors you should also have an alternate indoor activity, an activity you can fall back on in bad weather. For example, if you choose to jog outside early in the morning before work, you may want to purchase a treadmill for use at home on days when it is either too hot, too cold or the weather is bad.

Alone or with Others: On the plus side, an exercise partner can make exercise more enjoyable and can help you get going and keep going on days when you might otherwise quit. On the other hand, a partner probably means that you have the schedules of two busy people to contend with and plan around, which can at times actually hinder your workout.

How Much Are You Prepared to Spend: For many activities, you will need little or no special equipment. For instance, walking outside only requires comfortable shoes; whereas, joining and working out at a fitness center can be relatively expensive.

Aerobic Exercise: How Hard?

Because cardiovascular fitness should be your prime concern, **the central part of your exercise program should be an aerobic (or cardio) exercise done regularly**. Additional stretching and strengthening exercises should be included as time allows – but never to the exclusion of the aerobic portion of your program.

An aerobic exercise program should be vigorous enough to condition the cardiovascular system but not so strenuous as to exceed safe limits. I define safe as an exercise pace that is "comfortable." What they mean is that if, for instance, you are jogging or walking briskly you should be able to converse comfortably with a partner. You should be breathing and feeling normally within ten minutes after you stop exercising. If not you are exercising too vigorously. Other signs that you are pushing too hard include difficulty breathing, feeling faint, or feeling weak – during or after exercising. If you experience any of these symptoms, you are exercising too intensely and you should cut back.

Some experts prefer a more quantitative definition. They refer to the beneficial yet safe exercise region as the "Target Training Zone," or TTZ, which is determined by monitoring your pulse. The idea is to raise your pulse through exercise to a specific range (the target training zone) and hold it there for an extended period to obtain a cardiovascular benefit. On this concept rests the so-called heart-rated theory of exercise, which relies on heart rate (or pulse) to establish the proper exercise intensity.

Aerobic Target-Training Zone

The **Target-Training Zone (TTZ) is a measure of aerobic exercise intensity**. Use the following procedure to calculate your individual target-training zone:

1) Calculate your **Max heart rate** = 220 minus your Age. (Your maximum heart rate is the fastest your heart can beat, and you definitely must exercise well below this level.)

2) Compute your **Max heart rate reserve** = Max heart rate – Resting pulse.

3) Lastly, calculate your **TTZ** pulse = (Max heart rate reserve multiplied by Exercise intensity level) + Resting pulse.

If you would rather not do the mathematics, you may determine your TTZ from Tables 9 and 10. But before that, you need to determine the exercise intensity level that is right for you.

Aerobic Exercise: Intensity-Level

Many exercise physiologists recommend the following guidelines:

<u>Low Exercise-Intensity Level</u>: This intensity level should be used by anyone over 50 years old, and by those starting a physical fitness program after many years of inactivity regardless of their age. People in this classification should begin exercising at 40 to 50% of their TTZ.

<u>Moderate Exercise-Intensity Level</u>: This applies to moderately active people who are under 50 years old and who, for example, have been walking two or three miles per day regularly. These men and women may begin exercising at 50 to 65% of their TTZ.

<u>High Exercise-Intensity Level</u>: This level applies to very active, well-trained, fit people under 50 years old. These individuals may exercise at 65 to 80% of their TTZ.

Keep in mind that these recommendations are aimed at the general population. In other words, they may not be right for you. Some people cannot raise their pulse, despite vigorous exercise, into their target-training zone. If you are one of these individuals, you probably have a maximum heart rate that is lower than average and so should disregard the target training zones shown here. Rather you should try to establish and be guided by a lower, more <u>comfortable</u>, more personal, exercising pulse range.

In addition, be aware that some blood pressure medications (such as beta-blockers) may lower your maximum heart rate and resting pulse. If you are taking blood pressure medication, consult your cardiologist for guidance before using the target training zone approach.

Age	Resting Pulse	Exercise Intensity (%)				
		40	50	60	70	80
20	50	110	125	140	155	170
	60	116	130	144	158	172
	70	122	135	148	161	174
	80	128	140	140	164	176
25	50	108	123	137	152	166
	60	114	128	141	155	168
	70	120	133	145	158	170
	80	126	138	149	161	172
30	50	106	120	134	148	162
	60	112	125	138	151	164
	70	118	130	142	154	166
	80	124	135	146	157	168
35	50	104	118	131	145	158
	60	110	123	135	148	160
	70	116	128	139	151	162
	80	122	133	143	154	164
40	50	102	115	128	141	154
	60	108	120	132	144	156
	70	114	125	136	147	158
	80	120	130	140	150	160

Table 9: TTZ: 20 to 40 years old

Age	Resting Pulse	Exercise Intensity (%)				
		40	50	60	70	80
45	50	100	113	125	138	150
	60	106	118	129	141	152
	70	112	123	133	144	154
	80	118	128	137	147	156
50	50	98	110	122	134	146
	60	104	115	126	137	148
	70	110	120	130	140	150
	80	116	125	134	143	152
55	50	96	108	119	131	142
	60	102	113	123	134	144
	70	108	118	127	137	146
	80	114	123	131	140	148
60	50	94	105	116	127	138
	60	100	110	120	130	140
	70	106	115	124	133	142
	80	112	120	128	136	144
65	50	92	103	113	124	134
	60	98	108	117	127	136
	70	104	113	121	130	138
	80	110	118	125	133	140

Table 10: TTZ: 45 to 65 years old

If you do use the target-training zone approach, your pulse becomes your exercise guide. In addition, after a couple of months of aerobic exercise a sure indication that you are rounding into shape, making progress, is that your resting pulse slows down somewhat – especially if it was relatively fast at the start. This is because well-conditioned strengthened hearts are more efficient and so beat more slowly at rest. Trained athletes often have a resting pulse of 50 beats per minute or lower, whereas the "average" pulse is 72 to 76 for untrained men and 75 to 80 for untrained women. Furthermore, understand that as you become more physically fit you will have to exercise more vigorously to get your exercising pulse rate into your target-training zone.

Example: Determine the target-training zone (TTZ) for a 40-year old relatively inactive woman with a resting pulse of 70, whose physician has approved her intention to start an aerobic exercise program.

Because she is relatively inactive but also relatively young, following the exercise-intensity level guidelines outlined earlier, she determines that she may start her exercise program at about 50 percent of her maximum heart rate reserve. She determines her (TTZ) as follows:

Max heart rate = 220 – Age = 220 - 40 = 180

Max heart rate reserve = Max heart rate – Resting pulse = 180 – 70 = 110

TTZ = (Max heart rate reserve multiplied by Exercise intensity level) + Resting pulse

TTZ = (110 x 0.50) + 70 = <u>125 beats per minute</u>

(Note, the exercise-intensity level was converted from 50 % to the decimal equivalent 0.50.)

Alternatively, the 40-year old woman could have used Table 9, where first she would search the far left side of the table and locate her age (40). Then from the four possible resting pulse selections she would choose (70); finally she would run her finger horizontally (to the right) until it intersects the vertical column headed by the 50 percent exercise intensity level where she would find her TTZ of 125 beats per minute. Because it is difficult to get an exact pulse during or immediately after exercising and this is not an exact science, she should convert her calculated TTZ into a TTZ range. In this case, for a 50 percent exercise intensity level her TTZ range would be about 122 to 128 beats per minute.

When you cannot find your exact combination of age, resting pulse and exercise intensity level in tables 9 and 10, an estimating technique called interpolation (which is beyond the scope of this book) can be used to calculate your TTZ – although it would probably be easier for you to just use the TTZ formulae and the mathematical procedure illustrated in the example.

Aerobic Exercise: How Often?

The American College of Sports Medicine recommends that an exercise heart rate of 60 to 90 percent of your maximum heart rate should be maintained for about 30 to 45 minutes three to five days per week to become reasonably fit. They also stated, "For most people exercising at the lower end of their heart rate range for a longer time is better than exercising at the higher end of the range for a shorter time." The United States Surgeon General recommends that people accumulate 30 minutes of moderate activity on most, if not all, days of the week. More recently, the U.S. Institute of Medicine suggested 60 minutes of moderate exercise every day. To confuse matters even more, many exercise physiologists favor the following exercise schedule:

<u>**Low Exercise-Intensity Level**</u> (40 to 50% of maximum heart rate reserve): People in this category (because of their age or lack of fitness) should work up to exercising 60 minutes per day at least five days per week. Despite the low intensity exercise level participants should achieve what exercise

physiologists feel is an acceptable – albeit minimum – level of fitness.

<u>**Moderate Exercise-Intensity Level**</u> (50 to 65% of maximum heart rate reserve): Men and women at this level should build up to 45 minutes of exercise per day at least five days per week to achieve a minimum fitness level.

<u>**High Exercise-Intensity Level**</u> (65 to 80% of maximum heart rate reserve): In this category, individuals should work up to 30 minutes of exercise per day at least five days per week for a minimally acceptable fitness level.

As you can see, in general if you exercise at the lower exercise intensity levels your workout should last longer. Moreover, the longer and more frequently you exercise the greater your fitness reward. How fit you become is really a matter of your age, your genes, how fit you think you should be – and how hard you are willing to work. **But don't overdo it**! Again, it is worth repeating, everyone should have medical clearance before beginning any exercise program.

Aerobic Exercise: Typical Workout

First, do not smoke before you exercise (or after for that matter); do not eat for two hours before you start exercising, and refrain from drinking any alcohol for four hours prior to beginning your exercise routine. **A classic aerobic exercise routine consists of a warm up, your main exercise, and a cool down.**

- Start with a three to seven minute warm up. Three minutes of stretching is sufficient if you are going to engage in a low intensity Group C exercise such as badminton; whereas a longer seven-minute warm up is better preparation for a high intensity Group A aerobic exercises such as jogging, cycling or stair climbing.

- Then move on to 30 to 60 minutes of your main aerobic exercise.

- Finish with a three to seven minute cool down period. Once more, if you are finishing a low-intensity exercise three minutes is enough. After a moderate or high-intensity aerobic exercise a seven minute cool down is more appropriate.

<u>**Warm up:**</u> Going from a resting state to a moderate or high-intensity exercise is a large jump. The warm up period gives your body time to bridge the gap and get ready for the more strenuous exercise that follows. Tension in your muscles and nerves is released; your large-frame muscles, ligaments and joints are stretched and put through their full range of motion; and your arteries and capillaries start to dilate as your heart beats faster and your blood-flow rate increases.

Begin your warm up by walking slowly and gradually increase your pace as you approach the end of the warm up period. Next stretch. **Never**

stretch cold muscles. Many stretches are based on yoga, where you start with good posture and then use your body weight to stretch your tissues. The following is a list of stretching exercises for your arms, neck, back and legs that are especially suited for warm up and cool down periods. Stretches (c) through (g) are illustrated in Figure 1. (Some of these stretches can be done toward the end of the walking segment of your warm-up.) Perform the stretches as described.

a) <u>Neck Swivel</u>: From a standing position, with your arms hanging loosely, rotate your head about your neck, five times clockwise, then five times counter clockwise.

b) <u>Shoulder Roll</u>: While standing, with your arms hanging loosely at your side rotate your shoulders first in a forward motion, then backwards. Repeat five times.

c) <u>Arm Pumping</u>: Again, from a standing position, raise your elbows to shoulder height. Pull your elbows and arms slowly rearward as you thrust your chest forward. Repeat five times.

d) <u>Side to side Stretch</u>: From a standing position, raise both hands over your head. Bend slowly from side to side. Repeat five times.

e) <u>Toe Touch</u>: Sit along a bench and place your right leg on the bench. Position your left leg on the floor. Lean forward and try to touch your right toe until feel a stretch behind your right knee and calf. Do not bounce. Hold for a count of ten. Repeat with left leg raised. (This stretch can also be done from a standing position by placing a leg on a chair.)

f) <u>Wall Push to Stretch Calves</u>: Stand about two feet from a wall. Then as you extend your arms forward lean into the wall. Keep both heels flat on the floor. Do not bounce. Hold this position for a count of ten.

g) <u>Quad Stretch</u>: Balance yourself by placing your left hand on a wall. Bend your right leg and move your right heel toward your rear end. Grab your right foot with your right hand. Pull very gently. You should feel mild pressure in your right quad (the front of your right thigh). Do not bounce. Hold for a count of ten. Repeat for the left leg.

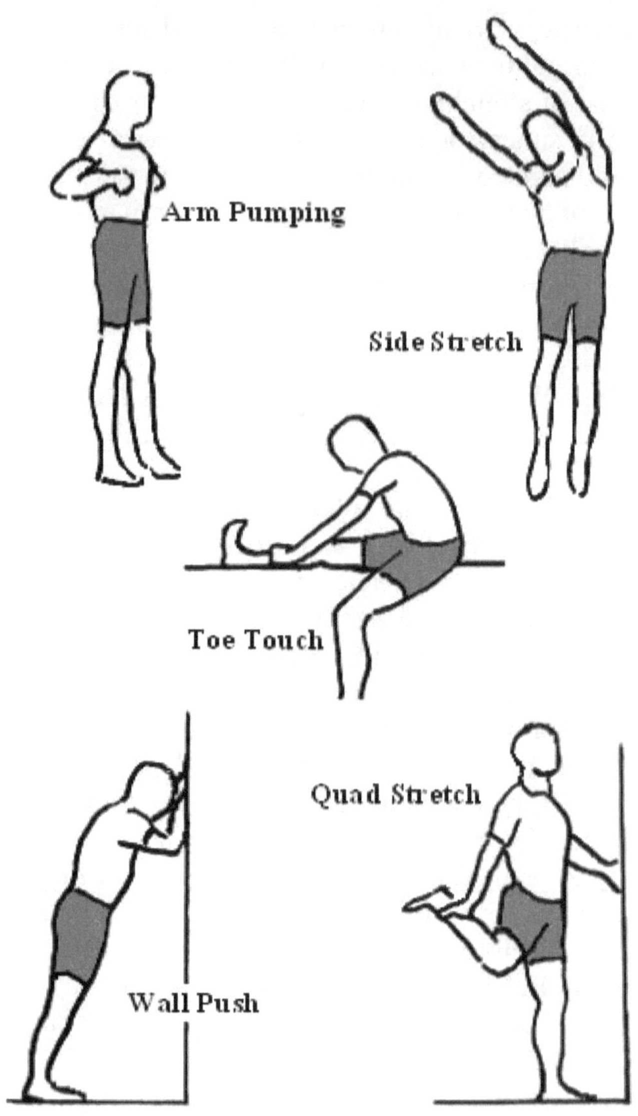

Stretching Exercises

Ladies, I apologize for using male figures to illustrate the stretching exercises. I misplaced the illustrations using female figures. They are being redrawn and will be available for the next edition of Total Fitness for Women. Thank you.

Do not feel limited to the preceding stretching exercises. There are many, many other good stretches available (too many to discuss here) that you might prefer.

If your main activity is a low-intensity exercise, you can conclude your warm up after stretching out. If you are going on to a moderate or high-intensity aerobic exercise, after stretching start your main aerobic exercise but at a relatively lower level. Over the next few minutes gradually increase the intensity so that your pulse approaches your target training zone. For instance, if you are a jogger you might warm up as follows: Start by walking slowly but steadily walk faster. After approximately five minutes stop and do two minutes of stretching. In theory, your warm up is over, but begin the main portion of your exercise by walking much faster, transition to a slow jog, then jog somewhat faster, and so on until, after about five minutes you have reached your regular jogging pace.

Main Exercise: Now you can begin your aerobic exercise of choice in earnest, stopping only to see that your pulse is in your target-training zone. If not, adjust your exercise level, exerting more or less effort. (Eventually, you will be able to sense that you are exercising at the correct intensity level and need only monitor your pulse occasionally.)

Cool Down: A five to seven-minute cooling off period should follow an aerobic workout. During cool down keep moving, decrease your activity level slowly. End your workout with leg stretches such as toe touches, a wall push and a quad stretch.

Pulse Measurement

In order to monitor the intensity of exercise, you should occasionally stop during your workout and take your pulse immediately. This is because your pulse will fall quickly once you stop exercising. The trick is to find your pulse within a couple of seconds and then start counting.

Quickly place the tips of two fingers on one of the two carotid arteries in your neck. (Your carotid arteries are located on either side of your throat.) Count the beats for ten seconds and multiply by six. For example, if you count 20 beats in ten seconds then your pulse would be 120 beats per minute.

You are doing fine if your pulse is within your TTZ range. If your pulse is too slow, exercise somewhat harder; if your pulse is fast, exercise easier. Again, after you have exercised for some time you will be able to feel that you are exerting the correct amount of effort and need only check your exercising pulse about once a week. (Note: The best way to find your resting pulse is to measure it immediately upon rising in the morning. Use the average over three days for the truest result.)

Monitors For Aerobic Exercise

The following are some other techniques and equipment you can use to measure and monitor the quality of your exercise regime.

<u>Heart Rate Monitor</u>: These devices track your heart rate by transmitting it to a Fit Bit, or a similar device you wear on your wrist. The monitor measures your exercising pulse and relieves you of that task.

Pedometer: Fastened to your belt or waistband, pedometers count steps, and once you determine your stride length a pedometer can also be used to gauge distance. Pedometers are relatively inexpensive. They are sometimes used in weight-loss programs – where people are advised to accumulate at least 10,000 steps a day (which is equivalent to walking about five miles).

G.P.S. Monitor: By determining your location, a Global Positioning System sensor can measure your speed, distance and pace during a workout.

Power Meter: Some cyclists use power meters to record power output, pedal revolutions, speed, time and distance. Most meters allow the data to be uploaded to a computer – but the meters can be expensive.

Walking Program

If your goal is to improve your general health and fitness, walking is a wonderful exercise. It's an exercise that you can do anywhere, that you can do outdoors or indoors, that requires no special equipment other than a good comfortable pair of walking shoes, and that you can do well into your old age. Walking does have a downside. Because it is a relatively low-intensity exercise, to get a good workout you have to spend more time walking compared to most high-intensity exercises.

If you are more than 50 years old, or have been sedentary for some time, it is best to start with a walking program that slowly but surely builds in intensity. If you walk hard enough, long enough and often enough, a walking workout can make you fit. A ten-week beginner's routine is shown in Table 11.

The first session in week 1 starts cautiously with approximately three minutes of warm-up walking at a very easy pace of about 2.5 mph. Continue your warm up with two minutes of stretching. (See the stretching exercises described in Figure 1.) Then start walking more briskly, about 3.5 mph, but you should check your pulse and increase or decrease this to get your heart rate to a TTZ corresponding to about a 50 percent intensity level. After eight minutes, start your cool down by reducing your walking speed again to about 2.5 mph for three minutes. Conclude your session by doing about two minutes of stretching. The total workout time in week 1 is 18 minutes per session. The only part that changes in succeeding weeks (2 through 10), is the brisk walking portion of the workout increases continually from 8 minutes in week 1 to 30 minutes in week 10.

Walk at least three days a week for ten weeks. If you find a week particularly tiring, backup to the previous week (or repeat the week) before continuing with the program. This is not a contest; you do not have to finish the program in ten weeks. Once you complete the ten-week program you can either stay on a walking routine, or go on to one of the more strenuous aerobic exercises.

Week	Warm up (Minutes)		Brisk Walking (Minutes)	Cool down (Minutes)		Total Minutes
	Walk	Stretch		Walk	Stretch	
1	3	2	8	3	2	18
2	3	2	10	3	2	20
3	3	2	12	3	2	22
4	3	2	14	3	2	24
5	3	2	16	3	2	26
6	3	2	18	3	2	28
7	3	2	20	3	2	30
8	3	2	23	3	2	33
9	3	2	26	3	2	36
10	3	2	30	3	2	40

Table 11: Walking Program for Beginners

If you decide to become a walker and want to improve, first go from walking three days per week to five days per week – at the same TTZ. To improve further gradually increase your total workout time from 40 to 60 minutes. To improve even more, gradually increase your walking speed, and TTZ, so that your exercise intensity level approaches 60 percent. Another good way to increase the intensity of your walking workout is to include some hills in your route. Incidentally, as you would expect, walking over hilly terrain also burns more calories than walking on level ground. On the two days you don't walk, try to get in 20 minutes of strengthening exercises.

Because you will undoubtedly do most of your walking outside, you have to be aware of the weather forecast and have a backup plan for inclement weather. On bad-weather days, you could use an indoor walking site (like a mall, or an indoor track), walk on a treadmill, or do stretching or strength exercises instead of walking.

Get a Pedometer and Step Out

Sedentary people only take about 2,000 to 3,000 steps a day. For the average person with a stride equal to about 2.5 feet (0.75 m), 2,100 steps amounts to walking about one mile (1.6 km). A Harvard University study has shown that 6,000 steps a day correlate with lower death rates in men, and that 8,000 to 10,000 step per day promote weight loss. And these health and weight management benefits don't oblige you to walk continuously until you accrue the required number of steps. Rather, all steps throughout the day to wherever and whenever count toward your daily total. (Some pedometers also show total "aerobic steps," correctly defined as those steps accumulated during at least 10 minutes of continuous walking at a rate of at least 60 steps per minute.) Because 10,000 steps a day may not be achievable by some people, particularly by those who are elderly, sedentary, or who have chronic diseases, rather than insisting on a blanket 10,000 steps per day, a stepping goal should be based on an individual's baseline steps plus an increment of additional steps. (Your baseline is the number of steps taken in an average day.)

A pedometer keeps track of your steps. And a study by the American College of Sports Medicine found that participants who used pedometers were motivated to add about 2,000 steps to their daily routine. To start a stepping program, buy a pedometer. Wear the pedometer for a week and determine the number of steps you take on an average day. This is your baseline. Then add the equivalent of half an hour of walking to your day, or roughly 2,500 extra steps per day. For example, consider a woman who wears a pedometer and notes that on an average day she accumulates 3,500 steps. Her goal should be to add the equivalent of a half hour of walking to her day, or roughly 2,500 more steps per day, for a daily total of 6,000 steps.

There are many little ways to add steps to your day, such as taking stairs rather than an elevator, parking further from your destination, pacing as you talk on the telephone, marching-in-place for a minute once every hour – and of course taking short walks whenever you can. So buy a pedometer – get off the couch and step out for your health!

Pedometer Calibration: Because pedometers count steps, to display the distance walked, you have to measure and then input your average step length. To do this walk a known distance with your pedometer in place and then divide the known distance by the number of steps. Generally, the longer the distance the more accurate the calibration. A local high school football field is a good calibration site, with a known 100 yards (300 feet) from goal line to goal line. In this case, to determine your average step length, divide 300 feet by the number of steps. (Let's assume your pedometer indicated it took you 113 steps to cover the 300 feet. Then your average step length is 300 feet divided by 113 steps which equals 2.65 feet. To input most pedometers, however, you will have to convert this to 2' 8".)

Jogging Program

If you are in reasonably good condition, have completed the "Walking Program for Beginners," or have been walking regularly, and have medical clearance, you can start a jogging program. Table 12 illustrates a 13-week beginner's schedule. Try to get your pulse into your TTZ but don't overdue it. Gradually, over time, you want to increase both the intensity and distance of your jogging routine. However, if you don't have the physical makeup to do both, always choose endurance over intensity; i.e., choose distance rather than speed, choose to jog longer rather than faster.

The first session in week 1 starts with approximately five minutes of walking at an easy pace of about 2.5 mph. Continue your warm up with two minutes of stretching. Then start walking more briskly, about 3.5 mph, but check your pulse and increase or decrease this to get your heart rate close to a TTZ that is roughly consistent with a 45 percent intensity level. After five minutes of brisk walking, jog for three minutes at a slightly higher heart rate, corresponding to about a 55 percent intensity level. Follow this with another five minutes of brisk walking and a three-minute jog. Cool down by walking again but now at an easy speed of about 2.5 mph for three minutes. Conclude your session by doing about two minutes of stretching. The total workout time in week 1 is 26 minutes per session. In weeks 2 through 13, the time allotted to brisk walking decreases as the jogging time gradually increases.

Jog at least three days a week for 13 weeks. Again, if you find a week particularly tiring, backup to the previous week (or repeat the week) before continuing with the program. Once you complete the program, if you want to improve, first go from jogging three days per week to five days per week – at the same TTZ. To improve further gradually increase your total workout time from 30 to 60 minutes. To improve even more, gradually increase your jogging speed, and TTZ, so that your exercise intensity level approaches 65 percent. Another good way to increase the intensity of your jogging workout is to try to include some hills in your workout. On the two days you don't walk, try to get in 20 minutes of strengthening exercises.

Because you will undoubtedly do most of your jogging outside, you have to be aware of the weather forecast and have a contingency plan for inclement weather. On bad-weather days, you might use an indoor track, try an alternate exercise like jogging on a treadmill, or do stretching or strength exercises.

As always, stop exercising immediately if you experience tightness or pain in your chest, become lightheaded or dizzy, are severely breathless, lose muscle control or are nauseous. These are warning signs of over-exertion and you definitely should lower your exercise-intensity level. If you experience these symptoms, it is also a good idea to seek medical attention.

Be aware that the pounding your body gets from jogging usually takes its toll over time. Many joggers have recurring, nagging injuries, particularly to their legs and feet. If you begin to suffer chronic injuries, remember there are other high-intensity aerobic exercises for which your body might be better suited.   At that point, you might consider switching to cycling, a rowing machine, swimming, etc.

Week	Warm up (Minutes)		Brisk Walking & Jogging (Minutes)	Cool down (Minutes)		Total Minutes
	Walk	Stretch		Walk	Stretch	
1	5	2	Walk 5, Jog 3 Walk 5, Jog 3	3	2	26
2	5	2	Walk 4, Jog 5 Walk 4, Jog 5	3	2	28
3	5	2	Walk 4, Jog 5 Walk 4, Jog 5	3	2	28
4	5	2	Walk 4, Jog 6 Walk 4, Jog 6	3	2	30
5	5	2	Walk 4, Jog 7 Walk 4, Jog 7	3	2	32
6	5	2	Walk 4, Jog 8 Walk 4, Jog 8	3	2	34
7	5	2	Walk 4, Jog 9 Walk 4, Jog 9	3	2	36
8	5	2	Walk 4, Jog 13 Walk 4, Jog 13	3	2	27
9	5	2	Walk 4, Jog 15	3	2	29
10	5	2	Walk 4, Jog 17	3	2	31
11	5	2	Walk 2, Slow Jog 2, Jog 17	3	2	33
12	5	2	Walk 2, Slow Jog 3, Jog 17	3	2	34
13	5	2	Slow Jog 5 then Jog 17	3	2	34

Table 12: Jogging Program

Your Body's Muscles

Your body has approximately 650 muscles that account for more than half your body weight. (You also have about 206 bones.) Rather than pectorals, abdominals, deltoids, trapezius, latissimus dorsi, triceps, and biceps, you will probably hear health club members using abbreviated versions, i.e., pecs, abs, delts, traps, lats, etc. Many of these muscles are referred to in the "Strength Programs" section that follows immediately. If you want to know more about your musculature, pick up a Human Anatomy and Physiology text at your local library.

Strength-Building Programs

As good as aerobic exercises are, they contribute little to building upper-body strength. And strength training can increase your muscle mass, which tends to increase your basal metabolic rate – and helps you control your weight.

If you are a beginner interested in strength training it's probably worthwhile to start by joining a health club, where you can get professional instruction on the proper use of exercise equipment, from dumbbells to rowing machines, and where you can compare different exercise routines. Another possibility is to hire a personal trainer for a couple of sessions to get you started on a program personalized to your fitness level and to teach you correct exercise techniques.

Of all the many strength-building options, I personally prefer free weights (actually dumbbells) because they can be used at home. Working out at home has some significant advantages. First, your workout takes less time because you don't have to drive back and forth to a fitness facility; second, you have the flexibility of dividing your workout into small time segments to fit your day, whenever you have time, such as when the baby is napping, and of course working out at home is certainly less expensive.

You can workout in a bedroom, basement, garage, attic – anywhere you have extra space. A set of variable (adjustable) weight dumbbells and a small weight bench don't take up much room and are all you need for a home-based gym. (Bear in mind, **knowledge and the discipline to work out regularly are far more important than fancy equipment**.) Before investing in a set of weights and a bench, however, it may still be worthwhile to start by joining a health club. At a health club you can get expert instruction on the use of free weights. And you may find that you actually prefer to workout at a club.

But if you do decide to opt for the convenience of a home-based gym, that would be the time to purchase a pair of variable-weight dumbbells and a strong weight bench (that will not tip over) for home use. Rather than an entire set of weights, purchase just enough dumbbell weight so that you can do a military press five times.

The seven dumbbell exercises that follow comprise a total-body workout, suitable for beginners, that involve all the major muscle groups. When done consecutively without stopping a series of exercises is called a circuit. To start, use the same dumbbell weight for all the exercises, a weight that allows you to do 10 to 15 repetitions of the most difficult exercise in the circuit. For the first week do one circuit per training session.

Your goal should be two circuits per session, which should take you about 20 minutes (with a two to three-minute rest between circuits). When you are comfortable at this level you are ready to increase the dumbbell weight – but by no more than roughly 10 percent (or one pound minimum). The seven exercises are illustrated in Figures 2 and 3. Perform 10 to 15 repetitions of each exercise.

a) <u>Bench Press</u>: With your head and back on the bench, hold a dumbbell in each hand to the side of your shoulders, palms facing each other. Slowly raise the dumbbells extending your arms above your shoulders. Pause, then lower the dumbbells down to the starting position. The bench press primarily works your pectorals, triceps and deltoids.

b) <u>One–Arm Dumbbell Row</u>: Hold a dumbbell in your right hand, palm facing toward your right thigh. Stand to the right of your weight bench and place your left knee on the bench. Support yourself by putting your left hand on the bench. (Flex your right knee slightly and lean forward so your back is almost parallel to the floor.) Slowly pull your right arm up until your upper arm is parallel to the floor. (Keep your right arm close to your torso.) Pause and lower your right arm to the starting position. After you complete a set, stand to the left of the bench and repeat the exercise with the dumbbell in your left hand. Rows mainly work your latissimus dorsi and rhomboid muscles.

c) <u>Seated Shoulder Press</u>: From a seated position, hold a dumbbell in each hand to the side of your shoulders, palms facing forward. Slowly raise the weights over your head until your arms are straight. Pause, then lower the dumbbells to the starting position. The shoulder press mainly exercises your deltoids, trapezius, triceps, latissimus dorsi and rhomboid muscles.

d) <u>Curls for Biceps</u>: Stand with a dumbbell in each hand, your arms hanging loosely, with your palms to the side your thighs and facing straight ahead. Keep your elbows tucked into your side and slowly lift the dumbbells until they are approximately shoulder high. Pause and lower the dumbbells to the starting position. Curls chiefly work your biceps.

e) <u>Tricep Extension</u>: With a dumbbell in your right hand, assume the same initial position as in the one-arm dumbbell row. Slowly move your right arm rearward until it is nearly parallel to the floor. Pause and then return the dumbbell to the starting position without bending your arm. After completing a set, stand to the left of the bench and repeat the exercise with the dumbbell in your left hand. This exercise mainly works your triceps.

f) <u>Front Squats</u>: Stand with a dumbbell in each hand, to the side of your shoulders, palms facing each other (inward). Slowly bend your knees and lower your body until your thighs are almost parallel to the floor. Try to keep your heels on the floor. Pause and gradually raise your body by straightening your knees. Squats work your gluteus, quadriceps and hamstrings.

g) <u>Curls for Abs</u>: This is not a weight lifting exercise but is a useful part of any routine. Lie face up on a floor mat with your hands folded over your chest and your legs bent. Keeping your feet flat on the mat, slowly curl your torso up and toward your thighs until your shoulder blades are off the mat. Pause, then return to the starting position. This exercise works your rectus abdominis muscles – your abs.

Remember to do about five minutes of aerobic and stretching exercises before and after your strength exercises, and to workout two to three (non-consecutive) days per week. Why non-consecutive days? Because strengthening exercises work a muscle until it's fatigued, and a day off is needed for muscles to recover, repair and rebuild. And listen to your body to determine your level of exertion. Don't over do it!

A final word about breathing properly: Never hold your breath during weight training. This can cause your blood pressure to get dangerously high. Rather, breathe naturally and try to exhale during a lift.

Ladies, Again I apologize for using male figures to illustrate the following dumbbell exercises. I misplaced the illustrations using female figures. They are being redrawn and will be available for the next edition of Total Fitness for Women. Thank you.

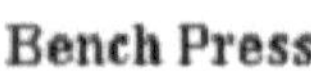

Bench Press

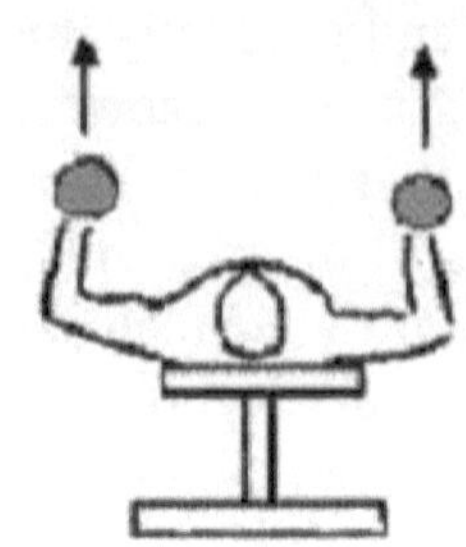

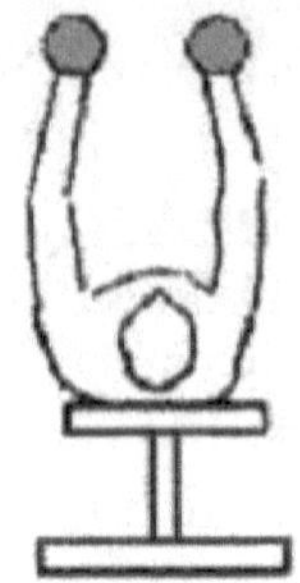

One-Arm Row

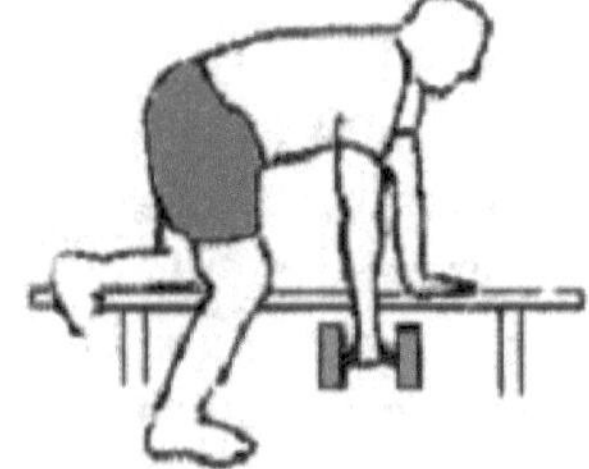

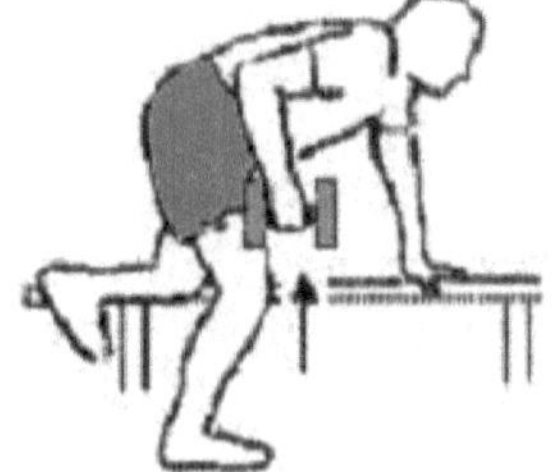

**Seated
Shoulder
Press**

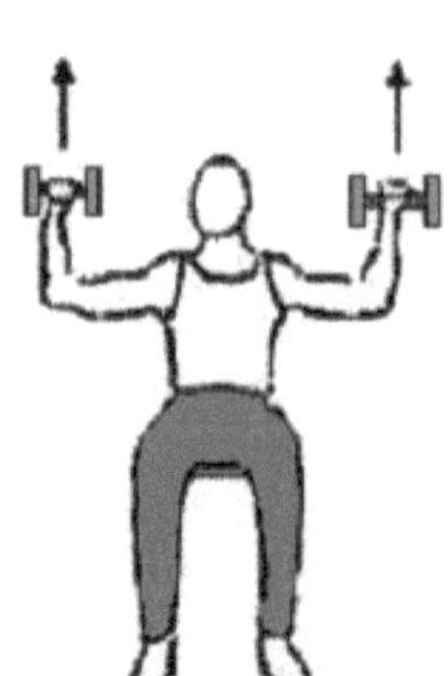

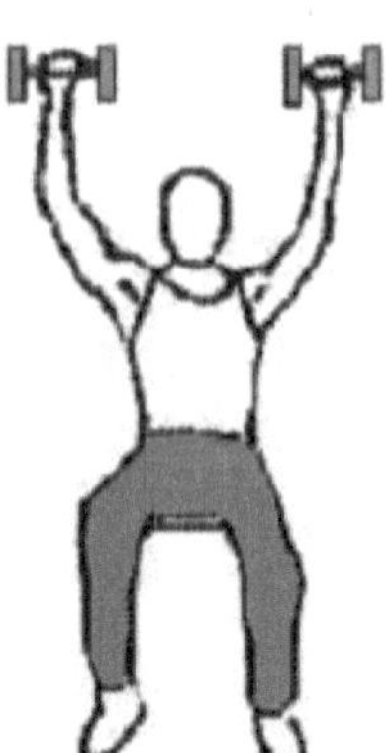

Strengthening Exercises (a to c)

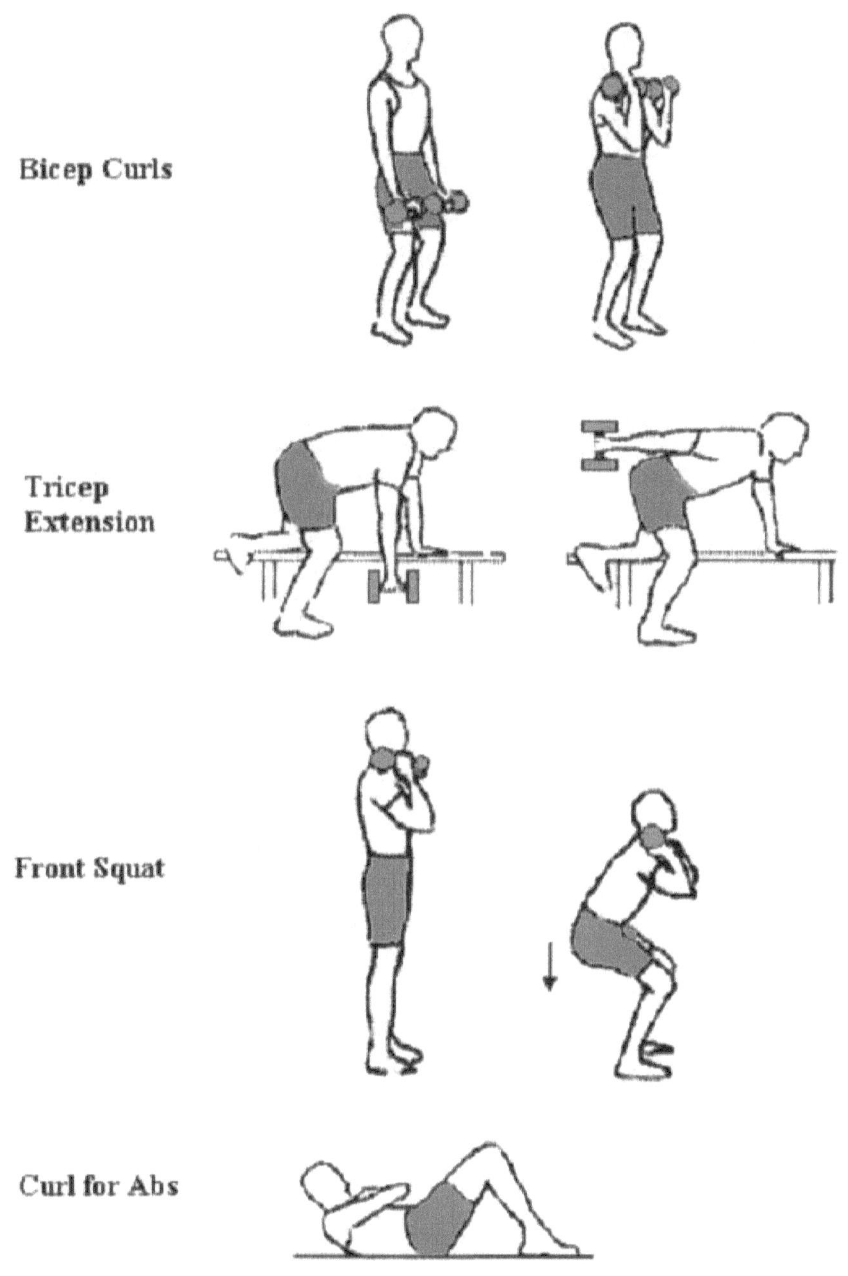

Strengthening Exercises (d to g)

Additional Strengthening Exercises

As your conditioning improves, you may want a more challenging workout. This can be accomplished in a number of ways. One method is to use two pairs of variable weight dumbbells, with a different weight loaded on each set of dumbbells. Now, you can more closely equalize the difficulty of the different exercises by using the lighter pair for harder exercises and the heavier pair of dumbbells for easier exercises. Yet another way to make your workout more demanding is to add one or more of the following exercises to your routine:

h) <u>Dumbbell Fly</u> (not illustrated): With your head and back on the bench, hold a dumbbell in each hand and fully extend your arms upward with your palms facing each other. Keeping your arms fully extended, slowly lower the dumbbells sideways to chest level. Pause, then return the dumbbells to the starting position. The dumbbell fly primarily trains your pectorals, triceps and deltoids.

i) <u>Dumbbell Pullover</u> (not illustrated): With your head and back on the bench, hold a dumbbell in each hand and fully extend your arms upward with your palms facing each other. Allow your arms to bend as you lower the dumbbells behind your head. Pause, then return the dumbbells to the starting position. The dumbbell pullover primarily works your triceps and deltoids.

j) <u>Standing Back Press</u> (not illustrated): Stand with your feet about 12 inches apart. Hold a dumbbell in each hand at shoulder height and slightly behind your shoulders, with your palms facing forward. Slowly raise the weights over your head until your arms are straight. Pause, then lower the dumbbells to the starting position. The shoulder press mainly works your deltoids, trapezius, triceps, latissimus dorsi and rhomboid muscles.

k) <u>Knee-Bend Kicks</u> (not illustrated): Sit on the floor and lean back supporting some of your weight on your forearms. Raise both heals about three inches off the floor. Flex and lift your right leg. Return your right leg to its starting position. Then do the flex and lift with your left leg. Repeat as often as you can. This floor exercise works your abdominals.

Other Exercises

There are literally hundreds of other aerobic, flexibility and strengthening exercises. Too many to review here, but many are definitely worth considering. For instance, swimming laps in a pool provides an excellent low-impact aerobic workout that also builds strength. Of course, the disadvantage is that you need to join a fitness facility that has a pool. Some trainers think a good rowing machine, such as the Concept II, provides a great total-body workout. Others feel a workout on a stairclimber is hard to beat. All have advantages and disadvantages.

In fact, most trainers recommend that you modify your routine every few months to add variety. Some advocate alternating exercises every other session. For instance, if you jog and lift weights on alternate days, you avoid repeating movements on consecutive days. As bonus, you will also most likely avoid the injuries that are often associated with day-after-day repetitive motion.

Missed Workouts

Inevitably, you will miss some workouts. It may be due to a heavy work schedule, a minor illness, or an injury. If you are injured or ill, wait for the injury to heal, or for when you feel like your normal self before resuming your exercise routine.

If you only miss a day or two, you can undoubtedly just pick up where you left off as if nothing happened. If you miss a week or more, however, you will probably have lost some of your fitness gains and might have to resume at a somewhat lower exercising-intensity level. This means that when you come back after missing some aerobic sessions, you might have to exercise at a slightly lower TTZ, or shorten the duration of your workout. And when you return after missing some strengthening sessions, you might want to reduce the weight you are lifting or reduce the number of repetitions.

Incidentally, physical fitness can be maintained only by regular workouts. If your exercise frequency drops to one day a week, half your fitness gains will be lost in 10 weeks. If exercise is stopped completely, virtually all your accumulated fitness benefits will be lost in five weeks! Therefore, if you want to keep that state of well-being, feeling better, looking better, it's important to make regular aerobic exercise part of your lifestyle.

Exercising in Hot Weather

When you engage in vigorous exercise, your body generates a great deal of heat, and your body temperature can rise from 98.6°F up to 101°F. (A body temperature of 105°F is life threatening.)

High ambient temperatures and high humidity are a concern because both influence how effectively you transfer the heat your body generates to the environment. High ambient temperatures are an obvious cooling problem, but high levels of humidity also cause cooling difficulties by hindering the evaporation of perspiration. As a result, on days when it is both hot and humid it is even more difficult to transfer heat from your body to the surrounding ambient air. This combination can cause your body temperature to rise to dangerous levels. **On hot humid summer days, therefore, you must guard against overdoing it**.

<u>Heat Index:</u> Adopted by the U.S. National Weather Service, the heat index, or apparent temperature, combines the effects of air (dry bulb) temperature and relative humidity. (Heat index values are expressed in either degrees Fahrenheit or Celsius.) The heat index is not perfect but it is the best guide for the general population. As expected, Table 4.6 shows that when the

heat index rises, so do health risks. In hot weather, the major health threats are heat stroke, heat exhaustion and dehydration.

Category	Heat Index	Heat-Related Risks
Caution	80 to 90°F	Unexpected fatigue possible with prolonged exposure and/or physical activity.
Extreme Caution	90 to 105°F	Muscle cramps and/or heat exhaustion possible with prolonged exposure and/or physical activity.
Danger	105 to 129°F	Muscle cramps and/or heat exhaustion likely. Heat stroke possible with long exposure and/or physical activity.
Extreme Danger	130°F or higher	Heat stroke likely.

Table 13: Health Risks in Hot Weather

Heat Exhaustion: As described in Table 13, when heat index values reach 90 to 105°F, you could suffer muscle cramps, particularly in your legs and heat exhaustion. The symptoms of heat exhaustion are pale clammy skin, dizziness or fainting, a rapid pulse, fast breathing, and nausea. If you experience any of these problems, get to a cool place, lie down and sip water. You may also need to seek medical attention.

Heat Stroke: Much more dangerous is heat stroke, which results when extremely hot weather triggers a malfunction of the body's thermostat, causing the body temperature to rise to 104°F or higher. Symptoms of heat stroke are confusion or loss of consciousness, flushed, hot and dry skin, a strong and rapid pulse. **Heat stroke is a medical emergency**. Move the person to the coolest accessible place and call 911. Some first aid measures include removing some of the person's clothing and sponging with cool water.

Dehydration: Everyone knows drinking water is important for good health, but it's even more important on hot days while you are exercising. During vigorous exercise, you can lose one to two quarts of water per hour in sweat, so it's essential to use common sense and stay hydrated. And in hot weather, drink plenty of water and fruit juice even if you don't feel thirsty.

Table 14: Heat Index

Relative Humidity (%)	Air Temperature (°F)									
	80	85	90	95	100	105	110	115	120	125
10	78	82	86	90	95	100	105	110	116	122
15	78	82	86	91	96	102	108	115	122	130
20	79	82	86	92	98	104	112	121	130	140
25	79	82	87	93	100	108	117	127	139	151
30	79	83	88	94	102	112	122	135	148	
35	80	84	89	97	106	116	129	143		
40	80	84	91	99	109	122	136	152		
45	80	85	93	102	114	127	143			
50	81	87	95	105	118	134	152			
55	81	88	97	109	124	141				
60	82	89	100	113	130	149				
65	82	91	103	118	136					
70	83	93	105	123	143					
75	84	95	109	128	150					
80	84	97	113	134						
85	85	99	117	140						
90	86	102	122	147						
95	86	104	127	154						
100	87	107	132							

Note: Exposure to full sun can increase the heat index by 15°F.

Another annoying problem in hot weather is chafing. Skin irritation can happen anywhere clothing touches your skin. If you are bothered by this troubling condition try different clothing styles, fabrics, or simply coat the affected area with petroleum jelly.

Before exercising outdoors in hot weather, check your latest local weather forecast. If the forecast does not incorporate the heat index, you can use the forecasted air temperature and relative humidity to determine a heat index value using Table 14. (Note the heat index values in Table 14 are in degrees Fahrenheit and the colors in the table correspond to those in the risk categories shown in Table 13.)

Frankly, unless you are relatively young and in very good physical condition, **it's not a good idea to engage in vigorous outdoor exercise when the heat index is over 90°F**. Despite this advice, if you persist on exercising on very hot days, make sure you wear loose-fitting, light-colored clothes; avoid the blazing sun (which can increase the heat index by 15°F) by working out early in the morning or in the evening; wear a hat and use sun screen; reduce the intensity of your workout; and drink plenty of water. In addition, be aware that the temperature of paved roadways can easily exceed 100°F even when the ambient air temperature is only 80°F. Therefore, if you are intent on jogging on hot days it's best to jog in a shaded park. Finally when you workout in very hot weather always let someone know when and where you will be exercising and what time you plan to return.

Exercising in Cold Weather

The ideal exercise temperature range is about 40 to 85°F with a wind speed less than 15 mph, but many people continue to exercise outdoors at temperatures well below 40°F. Generally, cold weather is less dangerous to an exerciser – but definitely not risk-free. When you exercise outdoors in cold weather you encounter an entirely new set of difficulties. Besides often-treacherous footing on snow-covered or icy surfaces, you must contend with low temperatures and the wind.

<u>Wind Chill Temperature Index</u>: Basic physics states that when heat leaves an object the temperature of the object drops. The same principle applies to your body. As heat leaves your body, your temperature drops and you feel cold. Very low ambient temperatures combined with the wind increase the amount of heat leaving your body. As the wind speed increases, the temperature of any exposed skin drops even further. The Wind Chill Temperature Index was developed in an effort to quantify this phenomenon, and is a measure of the relative discomfort due to combined cold temperature and wind. In essence, the wind-chill temperature lets you know what the outside air temperature "feels like," based on the heat loss from skin exposed to low air temperatures and the wind.

In 2001, the U.S. National Weather Service and Environment Canada jointly issued a new Wind Chill Temperature Index. Table 15 presents a version of the Wind Chill Temperature Index issued by the U.S. National Weather Service. (The wind chill-temperatures in Table 15 are in degrees Fahrenheit and the colors in the table correspond to those in the risk categories shown in Table 16.) Note that exposure to bright sunshine helps, because the sun can increase wind-chill temperatures by 10 to 18°F. The combination of low air temperatures and increasing wind speeds can result in incredibly low wind-chill temperatures. For instance, Table 15 shows that an air temperature of -30°F and a wind speed of 40 mph produces a wind-chill temperature of -71°F. Now that's cold! And dangerous!

Table 15: Wind-Chill Temperature

Air Temp (°F)	Wind Speed (mph)											
	0	5	10	15	20	25	30	35	40	45	50	55
40	40	37	34	32	31	29	29	28	27	26	26	25
35	35	31	27	25	24	23	22	21	20	19	19	18
30	30	25	21	19	17	16	15	14	13	12	12	11
25	25	19	15	13	11	9	8	7	6	5	4	4
20	20	13	9	6	4	3	1	0	-1	-2	-3	-3
15	15	7	3	0	-2	-4	-5	-7	-8	-9	-10	-11
10	10	1	-4	-7	-9	-11	-12	-14	-15	-16	-17	-18
5	5	-5	-10	-13	-15	-17	-19	-21	-22	-23	-24	-25
0	0	-11	-16	-19	-22	-24	-26	-27	-29	-30	-31	-32
-5	-5	-16	-22	-26	-29	31	-33	-34	-36	-37	-38	-39
-10	-10	-22	-28	-32	-35	-37	-39	-41	-43	-44	-45	-46
-15	-15	-28	-35	-39	-42	-44	-46	-48	-50	-51	-52	-54
-20	-20	-34	-41	-45	-40	-51	-53	-55	-57	-58	-60	-61
-25	-25	-40	-47	-51	-55	-58	-60	-62	-64	-65	-67	-68
-30	-30	-46	-53	-58	-61	-64	-67	-69	-71	-72	-74	-75
-35	-35	-52	-59	-64	-68	-71	-73	-76	-78	-79	-81	-82
-40	-40	-57	-66	-71	-74	-78	-80	-82	-84	-86	-88	-90

One of the **potential consequences of very low wind-chill temperatures is frostbite**. Table 16 (on the next page) employs the Canadian interpretation of frostbite risks rather than the U.S. version. (After all, who knows more about cold weather than Canadians?) **Other serious cold weather related conditions are hypothermia and heart attack.**

<u>Frostbite:</u> When body tissue freezes the injury is called frostbite, which usually strikes fingers, toes, nose and ears. Frostbitten skin is numb, hard and pale, and requires immediate medical attention. If you suspect you have frostbite, get indoors as quickly as you can and call or send for help. First aid steps include covering the frozen area with a blanket and drinking a warm nonalcoholic beverage.

Wind Chill Temperature	Frostbite Risk	Exposure Minutes
40°F to -17°F	Low	---
-18°F to -34°F	Medium	10 to 30
-35°F to -53°F	High	5 to 10
-54°F to -64°F	Higher	2 to 5
-65°F to -90°F	Highest	2 or less

Table 16: Frostbite Risk vs. Wind-Chill

<u>Hypothermia</u>: Prolonged exposure to extreme cold, especially during exercise, can result in a depletion of energy stores (calories) which can cause a drop in body temperature. This in turn can cause gradual mental slowing. The stricken person becomes increasingly unreasonable, clumsy, irritable, sleepy, and eventually lapses into a coma. This is a life-threatening condition. Severe hypothermia can lead to cardiac and respiratory failure and death. To help, your first move should be to call 911. Then start first aid (which is beyond the scope of this book).

<u>Heart Attack</u>: As the air temperature drops, your body's air-warming system may not be able to adequately heat the cold air entering your mouth and flowing down your windpipe. As a result, the incoming cold air may cause your coronary arteries to constrict – resulting in a heart attack – particularly if you are not in good condition.

<u>Upshot of Cold Weather</u>: Once the wind-chill temperature reaches about 10°F exercising outdoors becomes increasingly uncomfortable. Even if you are an outdoor enthusiast, at this wind chill you may want to think about changing to an indoor exercise routine until the weather moderates.

At a wind-chill temperature of about -17°F the risk of frostbite starts to increase. Unless you are skiing cross-country or downhill, or engaged in another winter sport that requires you to be outdoors, in bitterly-cold weather, the best advice is to exercise indoors. Furthermore, it is **not a good idea to exercise outdoors when the wind-chill temperature is below -20°F**. At this wind chill temperature any exposed skin will freeze in about 10 minutes.

In brief then, even if you are relatively young and in very good condition, rather than exercising outdoors in very cold weather, consider joining a health club, setting up a small workout space at your home, or walking in an enclosed mall.

Dressing for Cold Weather: Notwithstanding our best advice, if you still intend to exercise outdoors in frigid weather, wear layers of loose-fitting, lightweight, warm clothing. The layer closest to your skin should be a thin layer of a synthetic wicking material that draws perspiration away from your body. The second layer should provide insulation. Water-resistant fleece is a good option. Your third, outer layer, should be windproof and waterproof with a hood. Generally, mittens are warmer than gloves, and wool or polypropylene socks insulate and wick moisture. Wear a head sock that covers your entire head and neck with openings only for breathing and vision. Consider covering your mouth with a scarf to cause the air you breathe to be slightly warmer and more humid. Further, wear goggles or wraparound sunglasses to protect your eyes from wind and ultraviolet radiation. And make sure to stay dry.

In addition, remember to drink plenty of water – even in cold weather – to make up for water you lose when you sweat during vigorous exercise.

Exercise Risks and Problems

Certain situations may occur that indicate you may be doing too much, exercising too hard. For example, regardless of your pulse rate you should never be left completely breathless by your aerobic exercise. A good rule to remember is: **You are exercising too hard if you cannot carry on a conversation while you are jogging, cycling, etc**. A feeling of having worked hard is fine, sweating is good, but not a feeling of undo fatigue.

Perhaps the most frequent problems faced by exercisers are injuries of the joints and muscles: sprains and strains, knee pain, elbow pain, back pain, neck pain, shin splints and stress fractures. Most happen when you exercise too hard.

Potentially serious problems are signaled if you experience any of the following symptoms during or after exercise. The symptoms include but are not limited to any abnormal heart action such as an irregular heart rhythm; pain or pressure in the middle of your chest; pain in an arm or your neck; dizziness, fainting or lightheadedness; severe exhaustion; sudden loss of coordination; or confusion. If any of these symptoms are experienced, stop exercising immediately and get medical help.

Avoiding Injury

When he practiced, my friend Dr. Kanaar's specialty was rehabilitation medicine but he also preached what he called "preventive medicine," that is avoiding injury by practicing a common-sense approach to exercise:
1) Have a medical checkup and then set realistic fitness goals.
2) Build up your exercise intensity gradually over many weeks, months.
3) After you eat a meal, wait two hours before exercising.
4) Buy good suitable clothing for your exercise routine.

5) Use safety and protective equipment when appropriate, such as helmet when you bicycle, and goggles when you play handball, squash or racquetball.

6) On hot days, follow the precautions in the section "Exercising in Hot Weather."

7) On cold days, follow the precautions in the section "Exercising in Cold Weather."

8) If you insist on working out in very hot or cold weather, always let someone know when and where you will be exercising and when you are planning to return.

9) If you are new to a gym or health club, attend an orientation session before you use any unfamiliar exercise equipment. Otherwise, read the operating instructions carefully and ask someone qualified to help you.

10) For aerobic activities, warm up slowly to reach your TTZ and cool down slowly after you exercise.

11) Do not increase the difficulty of any activity (e.g., your walking or jogging distance, the amount of weight you lift) by more than 10 percent per week.

12) Jog on softer surfaces such as a level grass field, a dirt path, or a running track.

13) After exercising wait 30 minutes before eating.

14) As a final point, if you experience some early warning pain stop exercising.

<u>Minor Leg Injures</u>: Many minor leg injuries can be treated using the well-known **<u>R.I.C.E</u>**. method, i.e., rest, ice, compression, elevation.

- **Rest.** You may not have to avoid all physical activity; just take it easy.

- **Ice.** Apply ice for 15 minutes several times a day as long as there is swelling.

- **Compress** the area with a bandage or sleeve to help control swelling.

- **Elevate** the injured area above the level of your heart.

On the other hand, if early pain is ignored and you continue exercising, a minor injury may become more serious.

Keep an Exercise Log

Individuals who keep a record of their exercise generally exercise more often and have more success over the long term. How should you go about this? Keep an exercise log. A sample Daily Exercise Log is shown in Table 17 with one day filled in.

Day	Walking Distance	Time	Heart Rate	Strength Exercise	Dumbbell Weight	Reps	Sets
Wed 08/11	2.7 miles	45 min	122	Bench Press	10 lbs	12	2
	5522 steps			Rows	5 lbs	12	2
				Tricep Ex	–	–	–
				Press	10 lbs	12	2
				Curls	10 lbs	12	2
				Squats	15 lbs	10	1
				Abs	N/A	25	2

Table 17: Sample Exercise Log

A Fitness Expert's Ideal Exercise

A prominent 43-year-old professor of physiology was asked at the end of a speech to a group of business executives to give her definition of the "ideal" exercise. Without hesitation she reeled off her checklist, saying her ideal exercise would be one which:

- Is aerobic, preferably where the arms as well as the legs are used.
- Is efficient, yielding the maximum fitness return for the minimum time investment.
- Can be done every day if desired, outside or indoors, i.e., is not weather dependent.
- Does not require any special equipment or facilities.
- Requires only one participant.
- Is fun!

She went on to tell of her extremely busy schedule: laboratory research, classroom teaching, speaking engagements, consulting. Yet she said she exercised every day virtually without fail, whether teaching in Chicago, visiting her publisher in New York City, or speaking in St. Louis. She bragged that her total time expenditure on overt exercise was usually only 40 minutes a day.

Then she described the exercise program she now follows that she felt most closely met her ideal. She said she was a "morning person" and that she got in her daily exercise first thing in the morning. She warmed up by doing stretching exercises for a few minutes, and then while watching the morning news on television she jogged in place for 30 minutes – making sure her pulse reached approximately 145 beats per minute - high enough to put her at the 70% exercise intensity level. She did a few sets of push-ups, abdominal curls and finally more stretching as she cooled off. Then still perspiring she jumped into the shower, she would have taken anyway, toweled off and was ready for breakfast. She added that when she was home she also jogged in place, and for variety every other day she rode a stationary bike. She exercised every day.

In conclusion, she admitted that her real passion was tennis which she played whenever she could, but which she said was only an adjunct to her exercise program not the backbone. Her reason: She could not reasonably expect to fit at least three or four tennis workouts a week into her schedule. Arranging for courts and partners, driving to the tennis courts, changing clothes, taking a needed extra shower, the entire process took more than two hours per session. Besides, a good deal of the time she missed her tennis match because she was out of town or too busy to take the time!

My Personal Exercise Routine

I started jogging in the late 1960's. Of course I was much younger then. I jogged three to five miles almost every morning and worked out with free weights (dumbbells) on the days I didn't jog. After 20 years of jogging, the constant pounding resulted in a troubling number of chronic minor leg and foot injuries. So I switched to walking and I have been walking ever since. Now I'm a semi-retired senior citizen; so I have more time than most. For the past 15 years, from 6:00 to 7:00 am, I take a brisk walk covering slightly less than four miles. Most days I walk outside but when the weather is bad I head for a nearby shopping mall. For variety, every other day, I power walk in place for about 45 minutes using one of my six exercise DVDs to set the rhythm; then I complete my workout doing two circuits of the dumbbell exercises described earlier.

In warmer weather I golf (walk 9 or 18 holes) or hike (about eight miles) two or three times a week. On those days – that's my workout. Although just a week before this writing, I finished my brisk one-hour morning walk followed by 20 minutes of dumbbell exercises. Then later in the day a friend called and next thing I know I'm playing 18 holes of golf. Walking – of course. In total, I exercised 5 hours and 45 minutes, burned about 2000 Calories, and felt strong, definitely not tired, at the end of the day. Not bad for a senior!

In summary, one day I walk outside for an hour; the following day I power walk in place for 40 minutes using an exercise DVD and also lift weights; the next day I'm back to walking outside again; and so on. I've been doing this for 15 years. I exercise every day without fail. Every day! And because walking is the central part of my program, I almost never suffer an exercise-related injury.

My exercise routine combined with a sensible diet have kept me trim over the years (within three pounds of my college-graduation weight). Most people think I'm much younger than my chronological age – and I feel great!

Workout to Stay Healthy

If your goal is a chiseled body with washboard abs and the endurance and strength of a triathlon athlete, you're reading the wrong book. Sure the aerobic and strength routines outlined here will help you get in shape, slim down and get somewhat stronger – but your body is not going to be transformed into the physique of a world-class athlete.

This chapter is about how you should workout to get fit so that you feel good and stay healthy. And you're not going to get fit just because you join a fancy health club with lots of high-tech equipment – if you only workout once or twice a week, or every other week. Joining a health club is great – if you use it consistently.

The words that describe our kind of workout are consistent, determined, steady, persistent, dogged, unswerving, gritty, single-minded. Get the point? In our kind of workout, you decide that you will workout at least five days a week; that an aerobic exercise will form the core of your workout, and that you will incorporate some strengthening exercises two days a week. After that, it doesn't matter exactly what exercises you choose, what equipment you use, or what facility you use. These are secondary factors. What matters most is that you exercise consistently. **To improve muscle tone and overall fitness, feel good and stay healthy, you should exercise at least five days per week, day after day, week after week, year after year – for as long as you are physically able.** Remember the key words: consistent, determined, steady, persistent, dogged, unswerving, gritty, single-minded. Consistent!

Of course, there's a bit more involved. To feel good and stay healthy, you must also eat properly. That's next in section - Nutrition Basics.

NUTRITION BASICS

In the opinion of many researchers the makeup of the diet eaten by the majority of people in the United States is the single most important factor, albeit not the only one, accounting for our high incidence of death from coronary heart disease and stroke. It's no coincidence that accompanying the high mortality numbers is an increase in the amount of fat we eat, an increase in the number of calories consumed per capita, and the inevitable increase in the average weight of our citizens. All are directly attributable to our diet.

Healthy eating habits, the result of sensible nutritional practices, must be an integral part of any physical fitness program. In this chapter you will learn how to improve the "nutritional quality" of the food you eat, and, as expected, we will also point out foods that you should avoid, i.e., those foods that are loaded with "nutritionally-empty calories."

Our Disastrous Eating Habits

Food is far more than just an energy source. Foods are made up of seven basic constituents: carbohydrates, proteins, fats, vitamins, minerals, fiber and water. (Some nutritionists would add phytochemicals to this list – but more on this later.) For a healthy body you need to eat the correct quantity and proportion of all these components. You need protein, carbohydrates and fats, for growth, repair and energy. You need vitamins and minerals, albeit in relatively small quantities, so they can perform their vital roles in the thousands of biochemical reactions in your body. Fiber, the broad name given to the things you eat that your bodies cannot digest, is needed to assist your digestive system.

Fortunately, supermarkets have all the foods needed – and in abundance. Yet most nutritionists agree that a great many Americans are not eating well enough to sustain good health. In general, our diet is too high in fat – with an average of 40 percent of our calories from fat - contributing to atherosclerosis. Another culprit is sugar. As a nation we consume more than 100 pounds of sugar per year per person, totaling an unhealthy, nutritionally empty, 500 Calories per day. This large intake of sugar leads to obvious ills, such as obesity and tooth decay.

Add to this the increased use of processed and convenience foods, the proliferation of nutritional misinformation and deceptive advertising, and it is clear that we most people must improve their understanding of nutrition in order to eat properly.

Nutrients, Micronutrients etc

Before we begin let us define some terms. Nutrients and micronutrients are the components of foods that are essential to human life. Proteins, carbohydrates and fats are nutrients. Some nutritionists refer to. proteins, carbohydrates and fats as "macronutrients," and call vitamins and minerals "micronutrients" because they are present in foods in much smaller amounts than macronutrients. More recently, a new grouping of naturally occurring plant-based chemicals, called phytochemicals, or phytonutrients by some nutritionists, have been identified as having many healthful qualities, but unlike traditional macronutrients and micronutrients, phytonutrients are not needed by humans to live; i.e., their absence will not necessarily result in metabolic problems, or a deficiency disease.

In the sections that follow we will discuss proteins, carbohydrates, fats, vitamins and minerals, and phytonutrients in some detail.

Proteins are Building Blocks

Proteins are molecules of amino acids that are required for cell maintenance and repair, as well as for the regulation of a wide range of bodily functions. Humans need 22 amino acids in order to live. Our bodies can make 14 of the amino acids on their own, but eight of them, named the essential-amino acids, must be acquired from the foods we eat.

Some foods have all the amino acids needed to build other proteins. These are called complete proteins. Nearly every animal food, including dairy products, eggs, meat, poultry and fish are complete proteins because they contain all eight-essential amino acids. Soy is the only plant-based food that has all eight essential-amino acids.

Other plant-based protein sources lack one or more essential amino acids (i.e., amino acids that the body cannot either create, or manufacture by modifying other amino acids.) These incomplete proteins are found in legumes, grains, nuts, and seeds. However, consuming combinations of foods that have incomplete proteins can provide the same complete protein end effect as animal protein. For a complete-protein meal, simply eat any of the incomplete proteins with another but different incomplete protein, such as eating legumes with grains, or legumes with nuts or seeds, or grains with nuts or seeds. Examples of some healthy plant-protein combinations (that provide complete protein) are pasta and beans, rice and lentils, corn and beans, bean soup with whole-grain bread, split-pea soup with whole-grain bread, peanut butter on whole-grain bread, and tortillas with refried beans.

Around the world, millions of people do not get enough protein. Protein malnutrition can cause growth failure, loss of muscle mass, decreased immunity, weakening of the heart and respiratory system, and in some cases death. Whereas, in the United States and other developed countries, getting the minimum daily requirement of protein is usually not a problem, because almost any reasonable diet will provide most of us with sufficient protein.

Adults need about 0.79 grams of protein for every kilogram of body weight per day to keep from slowly breaking down their own tissue. (That translates as approximately 0.36 grams of protein for every pound of body weight.) A case in point, an adult weighing 154 pounds (70 kg) requires about (154 x 0.36), or 55 grams of protein per day. How much protein is in food? A few examples: There are approximately seven grams of protein per ounce of beef, poultry, fish, cheese or peanuts. Soybeans pack 10 grams of protein per ounce. Most other beans and lentils contain about six grams of protein per ounce. There are roughly three grams of protein in an ounce of whole-grain cereal, and milk has one gram of protein per fluid ounce.

Understand that foods are rarely straight protein. Some high-protein foods, such as marbled beef and whole milk, also come with lots of unhealthy saturated fat. Therefore, when you eat meat, eat the leanest cuts, and when you consume dairy products, choose skim or low-fat varieties. On the other hand, beans, nuts, and whole grains offer high-quality (albeit incomplete) protein with little saturated fat - but with lots of healthful fiber and micronutrients.

You Need Carbs

Carbohydrates provide your body with its basic fuel, the energy your cells need to survive. The staple of most diets around the world, carbohydrates provide essential vitamins and minerals, fiber, and numerous beneficial compounds (phytonutrients) that promote good health.

The simplest carbohydrate is glucose. Glucose, also called "blood sugar" and "dextrose," flows in the bloodstream so that it is available to every cell in your body. Your body's cells absorb glucose and convert it into energy to drive the cell. Glucose is a simple sugar, meaning that it tastes sweet. Some other simple sugars are sucrose, also known as "white sugar," fructose, the main sugar in fruits, and lactose, the sugar found in milk. They all taste sweet, and most are digested and enter your bloodstream quickly. When you eat fruit or drink milk, however, the natural sugar comes with vitamins, minerals (and fiber in the case of fruit); whereas the simple sugars in candy, for instance, are nothing but nutritionally-empty calories.

Then there are the more complex carbohydrates. Most grains (wheat, corn, oats, rice) and foods like potatoes, pasta and plantains are complex carbohydrates. In general, but not always, complex carbohydrates are digested more slowly than simple carbohydrates, and take much longer to enter your bloodstream. Most of us have heard that eating complex carbohydrates is good, and eating sugar-loaded foods is a bad. The reason is that simple sugars require little digestion, and when you eat a sweet food, such as a candy bar, or drink a can of soda, your blood glucose level rises rapidly. In response, your pancreas secretes a large amount of insulin to keep your blood glucose levels from rising too high. The large insulin response in turn tends to cause your blood sugar to fall to levels that are too low. As a consequence, about three to five hours after consuming sweets you feel lethargic and hungry. Many people react to this by eating yet another sweet, which can start a rollercoaster ride of surging glucose and then insulin. None of this is experienced after eating most complex carbohydrates, or a balanced meal, because the digestion and absorption processes are much slower.

Glycemic Index

Thinking of carbohydrates as complex or simple, as good or bad, is outdated. More recently, a system has been devised to classify carbohydrates. The system, called the glycemic index (GI), measures the effect a carbohydrate has on your blood sugar - quantifying how rapidly and to what level your blood sugar rises after you eat a food containing carbohydrates, compared to a reference food (usually glucose or white bread). For instance, a candy bar, which is digested rapidly has a high GI and causes an almost immediate jump in your blood sugar; whereas, lentil soup is digested more slowly and has a low GI. The factors that influence a food's GI are:

Fiber prevents the rapid digestion of the carbohydrates in food and slows the discharge of sugar into the blood stream. Higher fiber content results in a lower GI.

Coarsely-ground grains are digested more slowly and have lower GI values than finely-ground grains.

Less-processed carbohydrates, such whole-grain foods where the fiber, bran and germ are intact, are digested more slowly than highly-processed carbohydrates. It follows, therefore, that less processing usually results in a lower GI.

Unripe fruits and vegetables contain less sugar and have a lower GI than ripe varieties.

More acid or fat a food has, the slower its carbohydrates are digested and absorbed into the blood stream. More acid and fat in a food mean a lower GI.

These factors sometimes lead to unexpected results. For instance, some foods containing simple carbohydrates such as fruit have a lower GI than a complex carbohydrate like the potato.

The glycemic index uses a scale of 0 to 100, with foods that cause the most rapid rise in blood sugar having the highest values. In this book and many others, glucose is the arbitrary reference food, and is assigned a GI = 100. (For a given food, a GI less than 56 is considered low, a GI = 56 to 69 is medium, and a GI greater than 69 is high.) Note that foods that contain little or no carbohydrate (such as meat, fish, eggs, avocado, wine, beer and other alcoholic beverages) do not have GI values.

Glycemic Load

Some food scientists have come to recognize that a food's GI value alone does not provide enough information to judge how a particular food will affect your blood sugar. This is because the GI does not take into account how much carbohydrate is in a food serving, and your blood sugar level is influenced by both the quality of the carbohydrate (GI) and the quantity of carbohydrate you eat. With this in mind, researchers developed a new guideline called the glycemic load (GL) which takes into account both a food's GI and the quantity of carbohydrate the food contains. A food's GL is calculated by multiplying the food's GI by the number of carbohydrate grams in a serving. For a given food, a **GL less 11 is considered low, a GL = 11 to 19 medium, and a GL greater than 19 is high**. Most people consume 60 to 180 GL units per day, with a GL of about 100 for a typical diet.

Table 18 shows the GI and GL values for some common foods. Most of the data are from the on-line database of the University of Sidney (Australia). The difference between a food's GI and GL is illustrated by a simple example. Table 18 indicates watermelon has a GI = 72, quite high. In this case, however, GI alone is misleading because watermelon only has about six grams of carbohydrate per serving. (Watermelon is almost entirely water, with some fiber and a small quantity of carbohydrate.) So a typical serving of watermelon, has a GL = GI x (net carb grams) = 0.72 x 6 = 4.3, which is quite low. (Note in the calculation, watermelon's GI value has been converted from 72% to the decimal equivalent 0.72.)

Some diet book authors claim a food's GI and in some cases GL are the most important guidelines to use when planning a weight-loss diet. But consider the following: Pears (not shown in Table 18) are forbidden by some diets because of a relatively high GI = 40. However, a medium size pear weighing about four ounces has a GL = 4, quite low. Now consider a four ounce serving of peanuts with a much lower GI = 14, and an even lower GL = 2. For people on a reducing diet, based only on Glycemic Index or Load, a snack of peanuts appears to be a better choice than a pear. A medium-size pear, however, contains only 70 Calories, while four ounces of peanuts are loaded with about 650 Calories! Pears and peanuts are both healthy foods, but the extra 580 Calories in peanuts are certainly not going to help you lose weight.

The focus on a food's GI can lead to limiting healthful foods that may have a high GI by themselves, but when eaten in combination with other foods are not a problem. A nutritious baked potato may have a high GI, but

Food	Glycemic Index (%)	Serving Size	Net Carbs	Glycemic Load
Strawberries	40	1 cup (150 g)	3	1
Peanuts	14	3.5 oz. (100 g)	9	1
Peach	42	large (120 g)	8	3
Carrot	92	large (80 g)	4	4
Lentils	28	1 cup (150 g)	15	4
Orange	48	medium (120 g)	9	4
Watermelon	72	1 cup (120 g)	6	4
Apple	40	medium (138 g)	15	6
Ice Cream	65	1 scoop (50 g)	10	7
Bread (wheat)	73	1 slice (30 g)	11	8
Grapes	46	4 oz. (120 g)	18	8
Bread (white)	70	1 slice (30 g)	13	9
Corn (sweet)	59	1 ear (80 g)	16	9
Banana	50	large (120 g)	24	12
Oatmeal	58	1 cup (234 g)	21	12
Sweet potato	50	medium (150 g)	26	13
Spaghetti	45	6 oz. (180 g)	44	20
Potato (baked)	94	medium (150 g)	22	21
Rice (brown)	50	4.5 oz. (130 g)	48	24
Raisins	64	1 box (60 g)	43	28
Rice (white)	72	4.5 oz. (130 g)	42	30
Snickers candy	55	1 bar (113 g)	64	35
Glucose	100	(50 g)	50	50

Table 18: Glycemic Rank of Common Foods

when eaten as part of a complete meal is digested more slowly than its GI value would indicate. The main point is that if you use GI or GL values as the sole factor when selecting your food, you could be eliminating very healthy foods, and eating too many calories and often too much fat as well. It is important, therefore, to appreciate that a food's GI and GL numbers only allow you to evaluate how a food's carbohydrate content affects your blood sugar level. Because your body performs better when your blood sugar remains relatively constant, you should be aware of a food's GL rank and consider it when planning your eating pattern. But there are other important factors that must also be taken into account, such as getting the micronutrients you need from a variety of foods, including carbohydrates, and staying within your caloric allowance.

In summary, **carbohydrates are neither all good nor all bad.** Remember good carbohydrates provide needed micronutrients. You should try to get the bulk of your calories from the good carbohydrates, i.e., from fruits, from vegetables and from whole grains such as whole-grain cereal, whole-wheat bread, whole-grain pasta, whole-old-fashioned oats, brown rice, bulgur, millet, and hulled barley.

Cholesterol and Triglyceride Levels

Atherosclerosis has been linked to both blood cholesterol and triglyceride levels. Both fatty substances are found in the plaque on the walls of clogged arteries. There are two types of cholesterol: high-density cholesterol (HDL), the "good" cholesterol, and low-density cholesterol (LDL), the "bad" cholesterol. You should have your cholesterol and triglyceride levels measured during a regular medical checkup and should know and understand the readings. At this writing, the desirable readings for otherwise healthy individuals are as follows:

- **Total cholesterol: less than 200 mg/dl.**
- **HDL cholesterol: greater than 40 mg/dl.**
- **LDL cholesterol: less than 130 mg/dl.**
- **Triglycerides: less than 150 mg/dl.**

For people who have coronary-artery disease, most cardiologists insist that the total cholesterol level be less than 160 mg/dl and the even more important LDL cholesterol be less than 100 mg/dl. Recently, cardiologists have been urging patients with coronary-artery disease to reduce their LDL even further to below 70 mg/dl.

Often, cholesterol and triglyceride levels can be reduced by adhering to the eating recommendations summarized at the end of the section that immediately follows, called "Fats in Foods." Where a low-fat diet alone does not work, people with high cholesterol and or high triglyceride levels, may be prescribed cholesterol-lowering medication by their physician. For more information on this important subject, visit the American Heart Association website: http://www.americanheart.org.

Fats in Foods

Fats are found in vegetable oil, seeds and nuts, meat and fish, and dairy products, as well as in foods like potato chips and french fries (that are cooked in oil), cookies, cake, and so on. There are certain fats you absolutely need to survive (the essential-fatty acids), and others you would do well to drastically limit (saturated fats) or avoid altogether (trans fats). Chemically, all fatty acids contain carbon chains with hydrogen atoms bonded to the carbon, and all fats have the highest calorie density – containing nine calories per gram (more on this later).

Until recently, the best wisdom was to eat a low-fat, low-cholesterol diet. This advice is now largely out of date. The latest research seems to show that the total amount of fat in the diet may not be linked with disease. **What really matters is the type of fat in your diet.**

<u>Saturated Fats</u>: When all carbon bonds of a fat molecule are filled with hydrogen, a fat is said to be saturated, i.e., saturated with hydrogen atoms. Most saturated fats are animal in origin and are solid at room temperature (good examples are butter and the fat in meats). Generally speaking, you should avoid or at least severely limit your intake of saturated fats because they can raise both your total and bad LDL blood cholesterol levels which increases your chances of getting heart disease.

When hydrogen atoms are missing along the carbon chain the fatty acids are called monounsaturated or polyunsaturated depending on their exact chemical structure.

<u>Monounsaturated fats</u> (also called omega-9 fatty acids) are liquid at room temperature and are known as oils. They are "good fats" and are derived from plant sources, such as vegetable oils, nuts, and seeds. In studies in which monounsaturated fats were eaten in place of carbohydrates, LDL blood cholesterol levels decreased and HDL cholesterol levels increased. Monounsaturated fats are found in high concentrations in canola, olive and peanut oils.

<u>Polyunsaturated fats</u> are also liquid oils at room temperature and in your refrigerator. They are "good fats" and are derived from plant sources, such as vegetable oils, nuts, and seeds. Again, research has demonstrated that when polyunsaturated fats were eaten in place of carbohydrates, LDL blood cholesterol levels decreased and HDL cholesterol levels increased. Polyunsaturated fats are found in high concentrations in sunflower, soybean and corn oils.

<u>Essential-Fatty Acids</u> are class of polyunsaturated fatty acids that our body cannot create. These fats must be obtained from the food you eat. Essential-fatty acids promote absorption of the fat-soluble vitamins A, D, E, and K and are also thought to provide many disease-fighting benefits. Because essential-fatty acids are needed and our body cannot manufacture them, they must come from the food we eat. Essential-fatty acids fall into two groups: omega-3 and omega-6.

Omega-3 fatty acids are relatively hard to find. Foods high in omega-3 fatty acids are walnuts, tofu, flax seeds and oily fish (salmon, mackerel, sardines, trout and albacore tuna). Omega-3 fats are thought to be heart-protective. (The American Heart Association suggests that people with coronary-heart disease consult with their physician regarding the advisability of taking a fish-oil supplement.)

Omega-6 fatty acids, on the other hand, are more common, easier to find, and are in most oils including sunflower, soybean and corn oils.

Current thinking is that the consumption of omega-6 and omega-3 fatty acids should be in the ratio of 3:1, with about three omega-6 for one omega-3. Many Western diets, however, contain about 15:1, omega-6 to omega-3, which is not good for your health. Although you need omega-6, people generally eat too much of it and not enough omega-3 fat. The American Heart Association recommends that you eat fish (particularly fatty fish) two times a week, as a way to get a more appropriate quantity of omega-3 fatty acids in your diet.

Fat Type	Where found
Saturated	**Meat, poultry (especially the skin), dairy products, lard, coconut oil, palm oil, cocoa butter**
Trans Fats	**Fried foods, margarine, snack foods, commercially-baked cake and cookies, and fast foods**
Cholesterol	**Egg yokes, dairy products, organ meats, fatty and prime meats, poultry skin, shellfish (particularly shrimp)**
Polyunsaturated (Omega-3)	Mackerel, salmon, sardines, tuna, canola oil, walnuts, flaxseed, wheat germ
Polyunsaturated (Omega-6)	Corn oil, cottonseed oil, safflower oil, sunflower oil, soybean oil
Monounsaturated (Omega-9)	Canola oil, olive oil, safflower oil (hybrid), sunflower oil (hybrid)

Table 19: Fats in Foods

Trans fats are produced when a liquid oil is processed into a solid fat. The manufacturing process is called hydrogenation, or partial hydrogenation, and trans fats are an unnatural by-product. Partially-hydrogenated vegetable oils are considered especially unhealthy, because of the resulting trans-fatty acids and the added hydrogen saturation. Research indicates that trans fats are even worse than saturated fats because they not only raise bad LDL cholesterol but also lower good HDL cholesterol. Eliminating foods containing partially-hydrogenated oils from your diet is vital to good health.

In summary, it is becoming increasingly clear that saturated and trans fats, increase the risk for certain diseases while monounsaturated and polyunsaturated fats, lower the risk. The key is not to eliminate fat from your diet but to substitute good fats for bad fats, and at the same time try to reduce the total amount of fat consumed because all fats are very high in calories. The current scientific thinking regarding fat consumption is as follows:

1) Try to limit the total fat you eat to no more than 30 percent of your caloric intake.

2) Do not consume foods containing partially-hydrogenated vegetable oil because they are high in trans fats. This includes commercially prepared baked goods, snack foods, and processed foods, including fast foods. To be on the safe-side, assume these food products contain trans fats unless labeled otherwise.

3) Limit saturated fats, i.e., any fat of animal origin, to 10 percent of your caloric intake. Have meat less often, and when serving meat use lean cuts and trim the fat. Eat fish and poultry (white meat, without the skin) more frequently. Use fat-free or low-fat-milk dairy products in place of whole-milk dairy products. (Coconut and palm oil should also be avoided because they are saturated fats.)

4) When consuming fat, choose foods containing monounsaturated fats like olive oil and canola oil, and foods rich in polyunsaturated omega-6 and omega-3 fatty acids.

5) Try to balance your intake essential fatty acids by eating more omega-3 fatty acids, found in walnuts, tofu, certain seeds and oily fish such as salmon, sardines and tuna.

Vitamins and Minerals

The following is a listing of vitamins and minerals complete with a brief discussion of their function in your body, what foods supply the particular micronutrient, and the Recommended Dietary Allowance (RDA) – which is a reference number developed by the United States Food and Drug Administration to help consumers determine how much of a specific micronutrient a food contains. Summaries of the RDAs for vitamins are shown in Table 30 and minerals in Table 31. Notice that RDAs are frequently gender and age dependent, and pregnant and nursing women most often have special micronutrient needs.

Because of the rapid expansion of scientific knowledge regarding the role of micronutrients in human health, the U.S. Food and Drug Administration, in partnership with Health Canada, periodically assesses and updates the Recommended Daily Values. The following contains the recommended RDAs as of April 2006 for the vitamins and minerals discussed.

Vitamin A is a collection of fat-soluble compounds that play an important role in vision, bone growth, reproduction, cell division, and help prevent or fight off infections. Vitamin A also promotes healthy surface linings of the eyes, respiratory, urinary, and intestinal tracts, and also helps maintain the integrity of skin and mucous membranes. Using the long-established International Unit (IU) measure for the recommended dietary allowance (RDA), adult men and women need 3,000 and 2,330 IU (as retinol) per day respectively. However, the new RDA measure for vitamin A is the microgram (mcg), which translates for men and women as 900 and 700 mcg per day. Foods rich in vitamin A are orange-colored vegetables such as carrots, sweet potatoes and pumpkin; dark-green-leafy vegetables like spinach, collards and romaine lettuce; and orange-colored fruits such as mango, cantaloupe and apricots; and red peppers and tomatoes. One medium-size carrot supplies approximately 270 percent of your RDA.

Table 20: (RDA) for Selected Vitamins

Vitamin	Age					
	19-30	31-50	51-70	70+	Preg	Lact
A (mcg)	700	700	700	700	770	1,300
D (mcg)	5	5	10	15	5	5
E (mcg)	15	15	15	15	15	19
K (mcg)	90	90	90	90	90	90
C (mg)	75	75	75	75	85	120
B_1 (mg)	1.1	1.1	1.1	1.1	1.4	1.4
B_2 (mg)	1.1	1.1	1.1	1.1	1.4	1.6
B_3 (mg)	14	14	14	14	18	17
B_5 (mg)	5	5	5	5	6	7
B_6 (mg)	1.3	1.3	1.5	1.5	1.9	2.0
B_7 (mcg)	30	30	30	30	30	35
B_9 (mcg)	400	400	400	400	600	500
B_{12} (mcg)	2.4	2.4	2.4	2.4	2.6	2.8

Values for vitamins D, K, B_5 and B_7 are Adequate Intake.

Vitamin D is fat-soluble. Briefly, vitamin D is important in assisting the absorption of calcium, in forming strong bones and teeth and preventing deficiency diseases such as rickets and osteomalacia. For most adults, an adequate intake of vitamin D is 200 to 600 IU (which is equivalent to 5 to 15 mcg per day). In addition, your body can make vitamin D after exposure to sunshine. Good food sources include salt-water fish such as herring, salmon, sardines and fish-liver oils, as well as fortified milk and cereals. Small quantities are also found in egg yokes, veal and beef. An eight-ounce glass of fortified milk supplies about 25 percent of your daily needs.

Vitamin E is a fat-soluble vitamin that is a powerful antioxidant and acts to protect cells against the effects of free radicals, which are potentially damaging by-products of energy metabolism. Research is underway to determine if vitamin E, through its ability to limit the production of free radicals, might help prevent or delay the development of cardiovascular disease and some cancers. For adults, the RDA for vitamin E is 22.5 IU (as d-alpha-tocopherol) which is equal to 15 mcg per day. Foods rich in vitamin E are vegetable oils, nuts, seeds, milk fat, egg yolks, liver, dark-green-leafy vegetables, and whole-grain foods. Approximately 12 almonds provide 100 percent of your RDA for vitamin E.

Vitamin K is another fat-soluble vitamin, and is known as the clotting vitamin because without it blood would not clot. Some studies also indicate that it helps maintain strong bones in the elderly. Adequate intake of vitamin K for men is 120 mcg per day and for women 90 mcg per day. Good sources are dark-green-leafy vegetables, soybean, cottonseed, canola, and olive oil. People who eat these foods as part of a balanced diet should easily get enough vitamin K.

Vitamin C is a water-soluble, antioxidant vitamin. It is important in forming collagen, a protein that gives structure to bones, cartilage, muscle, and blood vessels. Vitamin C also aids in the absorption of iron, and helps maintain capillaries, bones, and teeth. The RDA for vitamin C is 90 milligrams (mg) per day for men and 75 mg per day for women. Foods rich in vitamin C are citrus fruits and juices, kiwifruit, strawberries, cantaloupe, broccoli, peppers, tomatoes, cabbage potatoes, and dark-green-leafy vegetables. A six-ounce glass of orange juice supplies 100 percent of a man's RDA.

Vitamin B is actually a complex of different water-soluble vitamins that often exist in the same foods. They perform an important role in our metabolism, in maintaining muscle tone along our digestive tract and in the health of our nervous system, skin, hair, eyes, mouth, and liver. The B complex vitamins are: vitamin B_1 (thiamine), vitamin B_2 (riboflavin), vitamin B_3 (niacin), vitamin B_5 (pantothenic acid), vitamin B_6 (pyridoxine), vitamin

B_7 (biotin), vitamin B_9 (folic acid), and vitamin B_{12} (cyanocobalamin). Many cereals are fortified with all the B vitamins. Depending on the brand, one serving of a fortified cereal provides from 25 to 100 percent of the RDA for all the B vitamins (except vitamin B_7 biotin).

Vitamin B_1 (thiamine) plays a vital role in the proper operation of your nervous system. Your body also needs B_1 to convert carbohydrates into sugar and then energy. The RDA for men is 1.2 mg per day and 1.1 mg per day for women. Vitamin B_1 is found in meat, wheat germ, whole-grains cereals and breads, in enriched cereals and breads, in beans, nuts and seeds, and in dark-green-leafy vegetables.

Vitamin B_2 (riboflavin) also has a crucial role in certain metabolic reactions, particularly the conversion of carbohydrates into energy. Riboflavin is also an important antioxidant. The RDA is 1.3 mg per day for men and 1.1 mg per day for women. The best sources of riboflavin are brewer's yeast, almonds, organ meats, whole grains, wheat germ, wild rice, mushrooms, soybeans, milk, yogurt, eggs, broccoli, and spinach. In addition, flour and cereals are often fortified with riboflavin.

Vitamin B_3 (niacin) helps clear toxic and harmful chemicals from your body. It also assists in the production of various hormones. Niacin improves your circulation and reduces blood cholesterol levels. The RDA is 16 mg per day for men and 14 mg per day for women. Foods containing significant amounts of niacin are liver, meat, poultry, fish, whole-grains and nuts.

Vitamin B_5 (pantothenic acid) is necessary for a variety of life-sustaining tasks such as generating energy from food, synthesizing essential fats, and the function of your adrenal glands. Adequate intake of vitamin B_5 for adults is 5 mg per day. Good sources include organ meats, eggs, fish and shellfish, poultry, soybeans, beans, dairy foods, avocado, and mushrooms.

Vitamin B_6 (pyridoxine) is needed for protein and red-blood cell metabolism. Your body also requires vitamin B_6 to make hemoglobin. For men and women up to 50 years old, the RDA is 1.3 mg per day. After 50, the RDA increases to 1.7 mg per day for men and 1.5 mg for women. Vitamin B_6 is found in a wide variety of foods including fortified cereals, beans, meat, poultry, fish, and some fruits and vegetables.

Vitamin B_7 (biotin) functions as a coenzyme in the synthesis of fat, glycogen and amino acids. An adequate intake of biotin is 30 mcg per day. A varied diet should provide enough biotin for most people. Liver, yeast and egg yokes are particularly rich food sources. It is also found in smaller amounts in fruit, meat and cheese.

Vitamin B_9 (folate or folic acid) helps produce and maintain new cells which is particularly important during periods of rapid cell division and growth such as in infancy and during pregnancy. Folate is needed to make

DNA and RNA, the building blocks of cells. It is also thought to prevent DNA changes that may lead to cancer. For most adults, the RDA of folate is 400 mcg per day. Of course, woman who are expecting or nursing need more folate. Cooked dry beans and peas, peanuts, oranges, dark-green-leafy vegetables and green peas are folate-rich foods.

Vitamin B$_{12}$ (cyanocobalamin) enables your body to manufacture healthy red-blood cells. It also assists in the transmission of electrical signals between nerve cells. The recommended dietary allowance is 2.4 mcg per day. Vitamin B$_{12}$ is found in fortified cereals, meat, fish and poultry.

Calcium is a mineral with several important functions. Most of the calcium in your body is used to support the structure of your bones and teeth. A small amount of calcium is in your blood, muscle, and the fluid between your cells. Calcium is also needed for muscle contraction, blood vessel contraction and expansion, the secretion of hormones and enzymes, and sending messages through the nervous system. For most adults, adequate intake is 1,000 mg per day. Foods rich in calcium are milk, yogurt, natural cheeses (such as cheddar, Swiss and mozzarella), canned fish with soft bones such as salmon and sardines, and dark-green-leafy vegetables. Eight ounces of milk (whole or skim) contains 30 percent of your RDA.

Chromium is important in the metabolism of fats and carbohydrates and in controlling blood sugar levels. It is an activator of several enzymes needed to drive numerous chemical reactions necessary to life. For men and women up to 50 years old, an adequate intake of chromium is 35 and 25 mcg per day respectively. After 50, the suggested adequate intake drops to 30 mcg per day for men and 20 for women. Whole grains, ready-to-eat bran cereals, seafood, green beans, broccoli, prunes, nuts, peanut butter, and potatoes are rich in chromium. One-half cup of chopped broccoli provides about 35 percent of your chromium RDA.

Iodine is a basic component of the thyroid hormone that regulates your metabolic rate. Lack of iodine can cause a number of physical and mental abnormalities. RDA for adult men and women is 150 mcg per day. Iodized salt, sea food and plants grown in iodine-rich soil are good sources of iodine. A three-ounce serving of cooked haddock contains about 125 mcg of iodine.

Table 21: RDA for Selected Minerals

Mineral	Age					
	19 to 30	31 to 50	51 to 70	70+	Preg	Lact
Calcium (mg)	1000	1000	1200	1200	1000	1000
Chromium (mcg)	25	25	20	20	30	45
Copper (mcg)	900	900	900	900	1000	1300
Fluoride (mg)	3	3	3	3	3	3
Iodine (mcg)	150	150	150	150	220	290
Iron (mg)	18	18	8	8	27	9
Magnesium (mg)	310	320	320	320	355	315
Manganese (mg)	1.8	1.8	1.8	1.8	2.0	2.6
Molybdenum (mcg)	45	45	45	45	50	50
Phosphorus (mg)	700	700	700	700	700	700
Potassium (mg)	4700	4700	4700	4700	4700	5100
Selenium (mcg)	55	55	55	55	60	70
Zinc (mg)	8	8	8	8	8	8

Values for calcium, chromium, fluoride & manganese are Adequate Intake.

Iron is an important mineral that aids the transport of oxygen in your body and is also needed for the regulation of cell growth. An iron deficiency limits oxygen delivery to cells, resulting in fatigue and decreased immunity. The RDA for iron is 8 mg per day for men and 18 mg per day for pre-menopausal women. Foods rich in iron are shrimp, clams, mussels, oysters, sardines, lean meats (especially beef), organ meats, turkey (dark meat), spinach, cooked dry beans, peas, lentils, and whole-grain breads and cereals. Three ounces of beef liver has approximately 50 percent of your iron RDA, and fortified cereals can provide from 50 to 100 percent of your RDA.

Magnesium is needed for hundreds of biochemical reactions in your body. It helps maintain normal muscle and nerve function, keeps heart rhythm steady, supports a healthy immune system, and keeps bones strong. The RDA is 420 mg per day for men and 320 for women. Dark-green-leafy vegetables, fish, some beans and peas, nuts and seeds, and whole grains are good sources of magnesium. One-half cup of cooked spinach has 75 mg of magnesium.

Phosphorus in combination with calcium is necessary for the formation of bones and teeth. Phosphorus is also involved in the metabolism of fats, carbohydrates and proteins, and in the effective utilization of many of the B vitamins. The RDA for adults is 700 mg per day. Rich sources of phosphorus are dairy products, meat, and fish. Phosphorus is also present in most soft drinks. Generally, a diet that provides adequate amounts of calcium and protein also provides a sufficient amount of phosphorus.

Potassium is involved in proper nerve function, muscle control and blood pressure regulation. (People engaged in vigorous exercise may need more potassium to replace that lost during exercise.) Low potassium levels can cause muscle cramping and cardiovascular irregularities. Adequate intake for men and women is 4,700 mg per day. Potassium-rich foods include baked white or sweet potatoes, cooked leafy greens, winter (orange) squash, bananas, oranges, dried fruits (such as apricots and prunes), and cooked dry beans and lentils. A medium-size baked potato contains about 600 mg of potassium.

Selenium is an essential trace element that assists enzymes involved in antioxidant protection and thyroid hormone metabolism. The RDA is 55 mcg per day for men and women. The most important sources in American diets are meats, fish and grains. Three ounces of cooked cod provide about 32 mcg of selenium.

Zinc is an essential mineral that stimulates the activity of approximately 100 enzymes that promote biochemical reactions in your body. Zinc supports a healthy immune system needed for wound healing, and helps maintain your sense of taste and smell. The RDA for zinc is 11 mg per day for men and 8 mg per day for women. Oysters contain more zinc per serving than any other food. Other good sources are red meat, poultry, beans, nuts, certain seafood, whole grains, dairy products and fortified breakfast cereals which can provide from 50 to 100 percent of your RDA.

Phytonutrients

Phytonutrients are not vitamins or minerals. Rather they are the beneficial compounds that give fruits and vegetables their many colors. "Phyto" comes from the Greek word for "plant," and that is where phytonutrients are found – in plant foods such as fruits, vegetables, whole grains, dried beans, nuts and seeds. Unlike traditional macronutrients and micronutrients (protein, fat, vitamins and minerals), phytonutrients are not necessary for life; i.e., they are not required for normal metabolism and their absence will not result in a deficiency disease. Despite this, research is expanding as evidence grows that phytonutrients have many beneficial qualities such as assisting the function of the immune system, reducing inflammation, acting directly against viruses, and playing a crucial role in preventing or reducing the risk of a number of chronic ailments, including heart disease, diabetes and cancer.

One of the most important roles of phytonutrients is as an antioxidant. Free radicals, which are by-products of energy metabolism, can damage cells and are thought to contribute to the development of cardiovascular disease and cancer. When antioxidant molecules encounter free radicals they neutralize them – limiting the damage. Our body needs more antioxidants as we grow older, because our body's ability to repair itself diminishes with age. Antioxidants are also thought to help prevent cell damage by environmental carcinogens.

Scientists understanding of phytonutrients is still in its infancy. Despite this, about one thousand phytonutrients have been identified to date and with ever expanding research new compounds are continually being discovered and organized into classes. The best known phytonutrient classes are carotenoids and polyphenols.

Carotenoids are contained in the yellow, orange, and red pigment in fruits and vegetables, as well as in dark-green-leafy vegetables (where the usual yellow color is masked by the vegetable's green pigment)

Some of the phytonutrients within the carotenoids class are alpha-carotene (contained in carrots); beta-carotene (in broccoli, sweet potato, pumpkin and carrots); beta-cryptoxanthin (in citrus fruits, peaches and apricots); lutein (in leafy greens such as kale, spinach and turnip greens); lycopene (in tomatoes, tomato paste, guava, pink grapefruit and watermelon); and zeaxanthin (in green vegetables and citrus fruit).

Polyphenol compounds are natural components of a wide variety of plants. Foods rich in polyphenols include apples, red wine, red grapes, grape juice, strawberries, raspberries, blueberries, cranberries, onions, tea, and certain nuts. Polyphenols are further subdivided into flavonoids and nonflavonoids.

Some phytonutrients in the flavonoids subgroup are anthocyanins (in fruits); catechins (found in tea and red wine); flavanones (in citrus fruit) flavones (in most fruits and vegetables); flavonols (in most fruits, vegetables, tea and red wine); and isoflavones (in soybeans). The nonflavonoids subgroup contains ellagic acid (found in strawberries, blueberries and raspberries).

Vitamin/Mineral Supplements

Even though most adults can get all the vitamins and minerals they need by merely consuming a variety of nutritious foods (from the fruit group, the vegetable group, the grains group, the meat and beans group, the milk group, and the oils group), **many physicians recommend a daily multi-vitamin/mineral supplement as a kind of insurance policy**.

Be aware that some micronutrients, such as the fat-soluble vitamin A, can be harmful if taken in large quantities. To be safe your multi-vitamin/mineral supplement should contain no more than 100 percent of the recommended dietary allowance (RDA) for each vitamin or mineral. Generally, you don't need the high doses in multi-vitamin/mineral supplements labeled "therapeutic" or "extra-strength." There may be medical reasons for taking larger amounts of a vitamin or mineral than the RDA provides, but check with your doctor first. For example, a physician may advise a pregnant woman to take an iron supplement, and women who could become pregnant to take folic acid in addition to consuming folate-rich foods to reduce the risk of some serious birth defects. Adults over age 50 and vegetarians who do not eat animal foods may be advised to get their vitamin B_{12} from a supplement or from fortified foods. Women with little exposure to sunlight may need a vitamin D supplement, and individuals who seldom eat dairy products or other rich sources of calcium may need to take a calcium supplement.

Dietary supplement choices include not only vitamins and minerals, but also herbal products and many other widely available substances. Herbal products, however, usually provide only small amounts of vitamins and minerals and their health value is currently being studied.

Guidelines for Healthy Eating

No single food can supply all the nutrients you need in the amounts you need. The most important factors in nutrition are variety, variety, variety! **Variety is the key to a nutritious diet**. As a means of setting strategies for food selection, the U.S. Department of Health and Human Services and the Department of Agriculture issue Dietary Guidelines every five years. The latest Dietary Guidelines recommend the following:

• **Make Half your Plate Fruits and Vegetables:** Eat red, orange, and dark-green vegetables, such as tomatoes, sweet potatoes, and broccoli. Eat fruit, vegetables, or unsalted nuts as snacks.

• **Switch to Skim or 1% Milk:** Both have the same amount of calcium and other essential nutrients as whole milk, but less fat and calories. If lactose intolerant, try calcium-fortified soy products as an alternative to dairy foods.

• **Make at least Half your Grains Whole:** Choose 100% wholegrain cereals, breads, crackers, rice, and pasta. Check the ingredients list on food packages to find whole-grain foods.

- **Vary your Protein Food choices:** Twice a week, make seafood the protein on your plate. Eat beans, a natural source of fiber and protein. Keep meat and poultry portions small & lean.
- **Choose Foods and Drinks with little or No Added Sugars:** Drink water instead of sugary drinks. Select fruit for dessert. Eat sugary desserts less often. Choose 100% fruit juice instead of fruit-flavored drinks.
- **Look Out for Salt (sodium) in Foods you Buy:** Compare sodium in foods like soup, bread, and frozen meals and choose the foods with lower numbers. Add spices or herbs to season food without adding salt.
- **Eat Fewer Foods that are High in Solid Fats:** Make major sources of saturated fats – such as cakes, cookies, ice cream, pizza, cheese, sausages, and hot dogs – occasional choices, not everyday foods. Select lean cuts of meats or poultry and fat-free or low-fat milk, yogurt, and cheese. Switch from solid fats to oils when preparing food.
- **To Maintain a Healthy Weight:** Basically enjoy your food, but eat less. Stay within your personal calorie limit. (Note that caloric needs will be covered in a later chapter.) Think before you eat: Is it worth the calories? Avoid oversized portions. Use a smaller plate, bowl, and glass. Stop eating when you are satisfied, not full.
- **Know your personal Daily Calorie Limit:** Keep that calorie number in mind when deciding what to eat. (Again, caloric needs will be covered in a later chapter.) Use a food log to keep track of how much you eat.
- **When Eating out Check posted Calorie Amounts:** Choose lower calorie menu options. Select dishes that include vegetables, fruits, and/or whole grains. Order a smaller portion or share when eating out. Cook more often at home, where you are in control of what's in your food.
- **If you Drink Alcoholic beverages, do so Sensibly:** Limit should be 1 drink a day for women or to 2 drinks a day for men.

Basic Food Groups

In this section we describe the various food groups, indicate what constitutes a serving size, and focus on the best foods within each group. (The foods in **bold font** are generally the most nutrient-dense foods – the best of the best.)

Fruit Group: Includes fresh, frozen, canned and dried fruits and fruit juices. Usually, a serving is 1 cup. A serving from the fruit group consists of 1 cup of fresh, frozen or canned fruit, or 1 cup of 100 percent fruit juice, or ½ cup of dried fruit. This group can be divided further into citrus fruits, berries and grapes, and other fruits.

Citrus fruits: There are many excellent citrus choices including **oranges, grapefruit, lemons, limes, kiwifruit and kumquats**. All are low calorie foods that contain a negligible amount of fat and cholesterol, are high in vitamin C, and most have significant amounts of vitamin A, potassium and dietary fiber.

Berries & grapes: Among the fruits in this grouping are **blackberries, blueberries, raspberries, strawberries, cranberries, gooseberries, purple grapes, black currents, raisins, and cherries**. Every fresh berry and grape is low calorie, with no fat or cholesterol, and all have small amounts of multiple micronutrients and a fair amount of dietary fiber. (Strawberries are also rich in vitamin C.) Some researchers claim that the blue and black-colored berries are packed with more disease-fighting antioxidants than any other fruit or vegetable. Of course, dark-red and purple grape contain the phytonutrient flavonol, the same antioxidant believed to give red wine its heart-protecting benefits.

Other fruits: This large subgroup includes a number of healthy foods such as **apples, apricots, bananas, cantaloupe, figs, mangos, papayas, peaches, pears, pineapples, plums, prunes and watermelon**. Again, most are low calorie, contain no fat or cholesterol, and are loaded with vitamins, minerals and phytonutrients. In addition, apples, apricots, figs, peaches, pears, pineapples, plums, prunes are good sources of dietary fiber. Cantaloupe is also high in vitamin C and watermelon contains the phytonutrient lycopene.

Vegetable Group: Includes fresh, frozen, dried and canned vegetables and vegetable juices. In general, 1 cup from the vegetable group consists of 1 cup of raw or cooked vegetables or vegetable juice, or 2 cups of raw-leafy greens. This group can be broken down further into dark-green-leafy vegetables, orange-colored vegetables, starchy vegetables and other vegetables.

Dark-green-leafy vegetables: Every food in this category (which includes **bok choy, collard greens, kale, mustard greens, romaine lettuce, spinach, Swiss chard and turnip greens**) is low calorie with no fat or cholesterol, and is packed with micronutrients, especially vitamins A and C, calcium, iron, potassium and folate, as well as dietary fiber.

Orange-colored vegetables: The best in this subgroup are **carrots, orange-bell peppers, pumpkin, sweet potatoes, yams and winter squash**. All have negligible fat and cholesterol and are high in vitamin A, potassium and dietary fiber.

Starchy vegetables: This grouping overlaps somewhat with the orange-colored vegetable subgroup and the grains group. Among the foods included are **white potatoes, sweet potatoes, yams, yellow corn, and brown rice**. These vegetables are generally high in complex carbohydrates, B vitamins, potassium and dietary fiber.

Other vegetables: This extensive category contains **asparagus, broccoli, Brussels sprouts, cabbage, cauliflower, celery, cucumber, fennel, green beans, parsley, and summer squash**. The preceding are low calorie foods that contain a negligible amount of fat and cholesterol, and most have significant amounts of vitamins A and C, potassium, calcium, iron, other micronutrients and dietary fiber. Also in this category are **eggplant, garlic, leeks, onions and mushrooms** which contain few calories, no cholesterol, and important amounts of potassium, calcium, iron and other micronutrients, as well as dietary fiber. **Red peppers and tomatoes** are low-calorie vegetables with no cholesterol that are loaded with vitamins A and C, iron and dietary fiber. Tomatoes also contain the phytonutrient lycopene. **Avocado and olives** contain some beneficial monounsaturated and polyunsaturated fat, but no cholesterol. Avocados are relatively high in potassium and vitamin A, while olives have significant amounts of iron and calcium.

Grains Group: Includes all foods made from wheat, rice, oats, cornmeal and barley, such as bread, pasta, oatmeal, breakfast cereals and grits. Generally, 1 ounce from the grains group consists of 1 thin slice of bread, or 1 cup of ready-to-eat cereal, or ½ cup of cooked rice, pasta or cooked cereal. <u>At least half of the grains eaten should be whole grains</u>.

Grains are the seeds of varied grasses grown for food. The outermost layer of the grain is an inedible husk, called chaff. The next layer is the bran, a protective coating rich in fiber. When this layer is removed, the product is described as pearled or polished. Inside the bran is the endosperm (the starchy part of a grain) and the germ, the part highest in nutrients (e.g., wheat germ). Whole grains have all these components intact. Refined grains have the husk, bran, and germ removed. Many foods are a mixture of whole and refined grains. Check the ingredient list for the words "whole grain" or "whole wheat" to determine if a food is made from a whole grain. In the United States, to be labeled "whole grain" a food must contain more than 51 percent whole grain by weight.

Whole grains include: **barley, buckwheat, bulgur, corn, millet, oats, brown rice, rye, wheat and wild rice**. Some whole-grain foods are: **whole-wheat bread, whole-grain ready-to-eat cereal, whole-wheat crackers, oatmeal, popcorn, whole-wheat pasta**, and whole barley (in beef-barley soup). All grains are low in fat and contain no cholesterol. Whole grains are good sources of complex carbohydrates and dietary fiber, as well as several B vitamins (thiamin, riboflavin, niacin, and folate), vitamin E, and minerals (iron, magnesium, and selenium).

Meats, Beans (and nuts) Group: Generally, 1 ounce equivalent from this group consists of 1 ounce of lean meat, poultry, or fish, or 1 egg, or 1 tablespoon of peanut butter, or ¼ cup cooked dry beans, or ½ cup of nuts or seeds. This group can be divided further into subgroups consisting of meat and foul, fish, eggs, beans, and nuts and seeds.

: **Skinless white-meat chicken and turkey** are relatively low calorie, low fat, low cholesterol foods that are powerful sources of high-quality protein, vitamin B_6, riboflavin, niacin, phosphorus and potassium. Most meats, even **lean meats**, are higher in fat and calories than chicken and turkey, but meats do provide high-quality protein and some important nutrients such as iron and B-vitamins.

 Most fish are good choices including **cod, halibut, herring, mackerel, salmon, sardines, scallops, shrimp, snapper, trout and tuna.** Nearly all fish contain high levels of essential-fatty acids. (Oily cold-water fish such as wild salmon, sardines, herring, mackerel and tuna are high in omega-3 essential-fatty acid. Trout also has comparatively high omega-3 content.) All fish are relatively low-calorie foods and are good sources of the fat-soluble vitamins A and D. (Fish-liver oils have high levels of fat soluble vitamins, and have been used as dietary supplements for many years.) Nutritionally, seafood is better known for its dietary minerals than for its vitamins. This is because some minerals in fish, such as iodine and selenium, are not available at the same levels in most other non-marine foods. Fish are also a good source of iron and potassium.

There is, however, a downside to eating fish. Some fish are contaminated with mercury, PCBs, dioxins and other environmental pollutants. Mercury is a toxic heavy metal that can accumulate in certain fish species. Large predatory fish such as shark, swordfish, king mackerel and tilefish have the highest concentration of mercury and other environmental contaminates. Canned white albacore tuna, a commonly eaten fish, contains higher levels of mercury than canned light tuna . The U.S. Food and Drug Administration advises adults to eat no more than six ounces of high-mercury fish per week.

PCBs are potential human carcinogens that find their way into fresh waters and oceans where they are absorbed by fish. A recent study reported that PCB levels in farmed salmon, especially those in from Europe, were about seven times higher than in wild salmon.

For further information about the safety of fish you catch locally, visit the U.S. Environmental Protection Agency's Fish Advisory website www.epa.gov/ost/fish or contact your state or local health department. If no advice is available, eat no more than six ounces per week of fish caught from local waters and do not consume any other fish that week.

According to the University of Michigan Integrative Medicine Department, pregnant and nursing women, and young children, should avoid shark, swordfish, king mackerel and tilefish, and strictly limit the amount of other contaminated fish consumed.

 Current dietary guidelines and the latest research concerning egg consumption appear to be at odds. On the one hand, because a typical egg yoke contains saturated fat and 300 mg of cholesterol, the latest dietary guidelines recommend that egg yolks and whole eggs be used in moderation (up to one egg per day), but that egg whites and egg substitutes can be used freely since they contain no cholesterol and little or no fat.

On the other hand, others argue that if judged as a whole food and not simply as a source of cholesterol, positives such as the fact that eggs are low calorie, are loaded with high-quality protein, are a good source of vitamin E, etc, are apparent. Moreover, researchers at the Harvard Medical School studied egg consumption among 120,000 nurses and other health professionals with normal cholesterol levels and reported no link between eating eggs and heart disease or stroke.

Some medical researchers advise that, if one is at low risk (i.e., does not smoke, exercises regularly, eats a healthy diet and has no family history of heart disease or stroke) and chooses to begin eating eggs, they should have a blood test four to six weeks after they start eating eggs to determine the impact on their total and LDL cholesterol. Based on the test results, your client and her doctor can decide – yes or no to her eating more eggs.

Beans: Among the foods in this important subgroup are **black beans, cannelloni beans, dried peas, fava beans, garbanzo beans, red kidney beans, lentils, lima beans, navy beans, and pinto beans**. All beans are inexpensive, low-fat, plant-protein-rich foods that are good sources of B vitamins, potassium, iron, dietary fiber and isoflavones (important phytonutrients).

Nuts and Seeds: This category consists of **almonds, cashews, hazelnuts, peanuts, pecans, pistachio nuts, walnuts, flaxseed, pumpkin seeds, sesame seeds, sunflower seeds**, and others. Because nuts and seeds contain significant amounts of essential-fatty acids, they are comparatively high-calorie foods. Most nuts and seeds have a good amount of dietary fiber, vitamin E, potassium, iron and folate. Almonds, cashews, peanuts, and pine nuts contain a significant quantity of plant protein and essential-fatty acids. Walnuts, flaxseed and pumpkin seeds are important sources of plant-based omega-3 fatty acids.

Soy: The soybean is the most widely grown legume. Healthful soy foods such as **tofu, soy nuts, soymilk, soybean oil, and soy protein** are made from soybeans. All contain a significant amount of plant-based <u>complete protein</u> and omega-3 fatty acid as well as vitamin E, potassium, iron and folate. Soy nuts are also high in dietary fiber.

Soybeans, tofu, and other soy-based foods are an excellent alternative to red meat. But there are some suspected dangers from too much soy. So advise your client not to overdo it. The Harvard University School of Public Health recommends two to four servings of soy foods per week as a good goal. Furthermore, they caution adults not to take supplements that contain concentrated soy protein or soy extracts, such as isoflavones.

Milk Group: Includes liquid milk and all products and foods made from milk such yogurt and cheese. (Foods that have little or no calcium such as cream, butter and cream cheese are not in this group.) In general, 1 cup from the milk group consists of 1 cup of milk or yogurt, or 1½ ounces of natural cheese, or 2 ounces of processed cheese.

Milk, yogurt and natural cheeses are high in calcium and protein. **Milk** is also often fortified with vitamin D. In addition to calcium and protein, **yogurt** is a particularly wholesome food providing live active bacteria cultures which promote gastrointestinal health. Choices should be fat free.

Oils Group: Includes vegetable oils and foods such as **nuts, olives, oily fish, avocados**, mayonnaise, soft margarine and some salad dressings. You should limit the intake of saturated fats – that is any fat of animal origin.

The oils group overlaps somewhat with many of the others. Liquid oils, however, are unique to this group. **Corn oil, flaxseed oil, safflower oil, sesame oil, soybean oil and sunflower oil** are polyunsaturated; whereas, **canola oil, olive oil and peanut oil** are monounsaturated. All these oils are high in calories and essential-fatty acids. Essential-fatty acids promote absorption of the fat-soluble vitamins A, D, E, and K. Flaxseed, canola and soybean oil contain omega-3 fatty acids. (Note, when purchasing olive oil, choose an oil that is labeled "extra-virgin" or "virgin." Virgin olive oils are produced from the first pressing of the olives, are unrefined and as a result are more healthful.)

Everyone should have a medical checkup before making major changes to their eating patterns. This is particularly important for anyone with medical problems and for women who are pregnant or breast- feeding, all of whom should consult a physician, nutritionist or registered dietician to determine the dietary pattern that is appropriate for them.

Calories, Calories

In order to plan a diet you must be able to estimate the calorie value of foods as well as portion sizes. The Nutrition Facts label on food packages, listing nutrient content, makes it possible to calculate the number of calories in a serving if you know that there are roughly:

	Calories per gram	**Calories per ounce**
Carbohydrates	4	110
Protein	4	110
Alcohol	7	200
Fat	9	260

<u>**Example**</u> Determine the calories in a cup (8 oz.) of whole milk. The label on a container of whole milk indicates that a cup has 11 grams of carbohydrate, 8 grams of protein and 9 grams of fat. The total calories in a cup of whole milk can be determined as follows:

        11 gm carbs x 4 Cal per gm = 44 Cal
        8 gm protein x 4 Cal per gm = 32 Cal
        9 gms fat x 9 Cal per gram = 81 Cal
        Total = 44+32+81 = <u>157 Calories</u>

A sense of the **caloric value (per ounce)** of some <u>basic foods</u> can be obtained from Table 22. The extremes of the chart are represented by water the lowest, at zero Calories, and fat (lard) the highest at about 260 Calories per ounce. Sugar (a pure carbohydrate) is near the middle of the ranking at 110 Calories per ounce . Protein is also approximately 110 Calories per ounce but there is no pure protein food to rank. (Note, most of the calorie values in Table 22 are the average of many varieties in a particular category.)

Water	0	Pasta	36
Coffee or Tea	1	Fish	42
Vegetables	7	Eggs	47
Milk (fat free)	10	Poultry	54
Soft drink	12	Whiskey	71
Beer	13	Bread	72
Fruit	15	Meat	97
Milk (whole)	18	Cake	100
Potato	23	Sugar	110
Corn	25	Chocolate	151
Wine	27	Nuts	175
Rice	33	Vegetable oil	253
Beans	34	Lard	260

Table 22: Calorie Rank of Basic Foods

Water	0	Peas	20	Liverwurst	79
Coffee or Tea	1	Yogurt (whole)	21	Hamburger	82
Vinegar	3	Potato (boiled)	23	Tuna (in oil)	82
Lettuce	4	Clams (raw)	25	Raisins	83
Celery	5	Banana	25	Bologna	87
Asparagus	6	Corn	25	Wheat Flakes	89
Tomato	7	Wine	27	Cake (average)	100
Spinach	7	Lobster	27	Sirloin Steak	103
Watermelon	7	Lentils	30	Cheese	106
Lemon	8	Scallops	32	Ham (baked)	106
Broccoli	8	Rice	33	Oatmeal	107
Mushrooms	9	Beans	34	Sugar	110
Cantaloupe	10	Pasta	36	Pretzels	111
Milk (fat free)	10	Tuna (in water)	36	Crackers	114
Carrots	10	Olives (black)	37	Doughnut	117
Strawberries	11	Blue Fish (baked)	45	Fudge	117
Green Pepper	11	Egg (boiled)	47	Chocolate	151
Peach	11	Turkey (light)	50	Potato Chips	162
Grapefruit	11	Ice Cream	55	Peanut Butter	167
Cola Drink	12	Sardines	56	Almonds	171
Beer	13	Turkey (dark)	58	Bacon	175
Yogurt (fat free)	13	Pancakes	64	Walnuts	180
Orange	14	Bread (wheat)	69	Butter	205
Apple	16	Whisky-86 proof	71	Mayonnaise	205
Milk (whole)	18	Apple Pie	73	Margarine	206
Cherries	19	Bread (white)	77	Vegetable Oil	253
Grapes	19	Jam/Jelly	78	Lard (fat)	260

Table 23: Calorie Rank of Common Foods

Table 23 is an expanded version of the Table 22 that includes the **Calories per ounce** of some commonly encountered foods.

If you appreciate that **most foods are some combination of water, carbs, protein, fat and fiber**, this can lead to a better understanding of why a particular food has the caloric value and rank shown in Table 23. For example, watermelon is almost entirely water, with some fiber (zero calories) and carbohydrate, with no protein or fat, and consequently has a very low 7 Calories per ounce value. A grape is again mostly water with some fiber and carbohydrate and according to the chart has only 19 Calories per ounce, but a raisin (a dried grape) is almost entirely carbohydrate and fiber with little water and thus has a value of 83 Calories per ounce – closer to the 110 Calories per ounce of a pure carbohydrate. When a food is not listed in the chart, common sense can often be used to estimate its caloric value; e.g., green beans are not listed, but judging from the ranking of similar foods a value of 6 or 7 Calories per ounce seems reasonable.

Table 23 can also be thought of as a listing of the "caloric density" of foods. For instance, the table illustrates that eight ounces (half pound) of carrots contains about 80 Calories, or approximately the same number of calories as one ounce of hamburger at 82 Calories per ounce. (Note that the numbers in the table are approximate Calories per fluid or dry ounce.)

Moreover, Table 23 in combination with a small weighing scale makes a very useful diet aide, allowing the calorie value of many food portions to be estimated quite accurately. It is a simple mater to weigh a piece of meat or a pancake, or a slice of apple pie, and multiply the weight in ounces by the calorie value per ounce (from Table 23) to determine the total number of calories. Frequently, this approach will result in more precise calorie values than those obtained from the numbers shown in a common calorie table where the portion size is often ambiguously described.

Estimating Calories in a Meal

As discussed, you must be able to judge the caloric value of foods if you are going to successfully control your weight. Another useful technique in this regard is to use an engineering-like approach. The first thing an engineer does when performing most calculations is to "ball-park" the answer. You will often hear an engineer remark, "Should the diameter of that shaft (for example) be one inch or ten inches? What ball-park are we in?" Initially he or she does a relatively crude, quick, over-simplified calculation that yields a "ball-park" answer. Later, time and circumstances permitting, the engineer will go back and do a more thorough analysis, considering all the subtleties of the problem. It is recommended that you approach calorie counting in much the same manner.

For example, you're having a meal with friends and you're served a concoction you hardly recognize. Try to dissect the ingredients on your plate and make a mental estimate the calories – so you can compensate by eating less the next day. Of course, you don't have access to an accurate calorie chart, and even with one (without knowing the exact ingredients of the recipe) you would be lucky to come within 50 Calories of the true total. In situations like this, don't waste your time trying to decide if that slice of bread you ate was 65 or 70 Calories, when your best guess for the main dish is 400 and 600 Calories. What you should do is make a "ball-park" estimate.

To "ballpark," first you must know what elements are significant and then what approximate value you should assign to these elements. In other words, first you must know what foods or ingredients are significant, that you should even bother counting, and then you assign an approximate calorie value to these foods or ingredients using Table 23 – which is designed to help you make quick and reasonable estimates.

You Need Fiber

Fiber is an important part of a healthy diet. **You need to consume fiber to assist your digestive system**. According to the Harvard University School of Public Health, adequate fiber intake reduces the risk of developing various conditions, including heart disease, diabetes, diverticular disease, and constipation.

Three fibers that are eaten on a regular basis are cellulose, hemicellulose and pectin. Hemicellulose is found in the hulls of different grains like wheat; e.g., wheat bran is hemicellulose. Cellulose is the structural component of plants, and gives vegetables their familiar shape. Pectin is found most often in fruits, is soluble in water but non-digestible, and is usually referred to as "water-soluble fiber." The best fiber sources are:

- **Whole-grain** breads, whole-grain cereals, whole-wheat pasta and brown rice contain a great deal of hemicellulose fiber.
- **Fruits** are pectin rich (the water-soluble fiber). The skin on fruits are loaded with phytonutrients and fiber. So do not peal an apple. Eat it with the skin on and get a fiber and nutrient boost.
- **Most berries** (such as bilberries, raspberries) have even more fiber than a comparable weight of most other fruit selections.
- **Vegetables** have lots of cellulose fiber. Again the skin is particularly high in fiber. When you eat a baked potato, eat it skin and all – everything – everything that is except the butter or sour cream.
- **Peas and beans** are high fiber foods that are also a complete protein when eaten with a whole grain food, or nuts, or seeds.
- **Nuts and seeds** add fiber to your diet.

When you eat fiber, in any of its forms, it simply passes straight through, untouched by but aiding your digestive system. Zero calories absorbed!

Adults should get a least 20 to 35 grams of dietary fiber per day. How much fiber is in the foods you eat? An apple has 3 grams of fiber, a tangerine has 2 grams, ½ cup cabbage contains 2 grams, a tomato has 2 grams, ½ cup broccoli has 1 gram, ½ cup of lima beans contains 4 grams, 1 cup of brown rice has 3 grams, 1 cup of whole-wheat cereal holds 3 grams and 1 slice of whole-wheat bread contains 2 grams of fiber.

Water, Water Everywhere

The average adult female body is about 52 percent water, while the average adult male is approximately 63 percent water. If you are average, everyday you lose about 10 cups of water when you breathe, perspire, and excrete waste. Because water is needed for almost every biochemical and physiologic process in your body, to maintain your body's water balance you must replace this lost water. (The water in your body is said to be balanced, when your water intake from all sources equals your loss of water.)

Typically, the food you eat every day contains about 3 cups of mostly concealed water. When you metabolize the food you eat, you create another cup of water. That leaves about six cups that must be replaced by the liquids you drink – even more when you exercise. It appears, therefore, that the long-established wisdom advocating that you drink eight glasses of water per day (or any other healthy beverage such as tea or fruit juice) is not far from the mark.

Use Salt Sparingly

Sodium and sodium chloride (salt) normally occur in small quantities in many natural foods. Salt and sodium-containing ingredients are also frequently found in high amounts in processed foods, such as canned soup and baked goods. People also add salt during food preparation and to the food they eat. Although sodium plays an important role in your body, many studies have demonstrated that high sodium intake is also associated with high blood pressure. In your body, sodium retains water expanding blood volume which in turn raises blood pressure. Moreover, although some questions remain, evidence suggests that many adults who are predisposed to high blood pressure (for example having a parent who has high blood pressure) can reduce their chances of developing high blood pressure by consuming less sodium.

Most Americans consume too much sodium. The U.S. Department of Health and Human Services and the Department of Agriculture Dietary Guidelines recommend that healthy adults **limit sodium intake to 2,400 mg per day.** (Note that one level teaspoon of salt contains about 2,300 mg of sodium.) Individuals who have high blood pressure and are also salt sensitive are frequently advised to limit their sodium intake even further.

Not Too Much Sugar

Sugars are carbohydrates that come in many forms. Sugar is found naturally in fruits, some vegetables, milk, breads, cereals and grains, and is often added to foods during processing, preparation and when eating. Added sugar and naturally occurring sugars are chemically identical and your body cannot distinguish between them. Cake, cookies, candy and many soft drinks contain large amounts of added sugar that supply a large number of "nutritionally-empty calories." Only very active people with high calorie needs can afford to consume any quantity of these sugar-laden foods. **Sugar should be used sparingly** by people with low calorie needs and in moderation by most other healthy adults. (Contrary to what many believe, the latest scientific evidence seems to indicate diets high in sugar do not cause diabetes. Rather, scientific evidence indicates that adult-onset diabetes occurs most often in those who are overweight.)

Common-Sense Nutrition

1) **Know your daily caloric allowance** whether you are trying to maintain your weight or are on a reducing diet.
2) **Eat a variety of foods** within your caloric allowance, and consult the **Basic Food Groups** on page 76 to shape your eating patterns. Try to choose the proper quantity from each food group.
3) **Try not to consume foods containing partially-hydrogenated vegetable oil** because they are high in trans fats. This includes commercially prepared baked goods, snack foods, and processed foods, including most fast foods.
4) **Limit your intake of saturated fats.** Eat meat less often and fish and poultry more often, and use fat-free milk and milk products.
5) **When possible, select fresh and natural foods and whole-grain products,** and avoid chemical preservatives and additives, artificial and imitation foods, refined and processed foods, and foods that are mostly "nutritionally-empty calories."
6) **Eat nutritionally-dense foods** rather than calorie-dense foods.
7) **Take a daily multi-vitamin/mineral supplement.**
8) Before you buy, **read and understand the labels on food packages.**

Eat Slowly

One final important point, try to **eat slowly.** This is especially vital if you are on a diet, trying to lose weight. If you are someone who eats fast, who finishes before everyone else at the table, you are not giving yourself a chance to feel full. While everyone else is still eating, you either sit there and pick, or you have seconds, taking in extra calories you could avoid if you would just slow down. To slow down, try eating smaller mouthfuls, try chewing your food more thoroughly, and try talking more at the table.

88

WEIGHT LOSS

All human life depends on the energy that comes from the sun. Plants convert solar energy into chemical energy by photosynthesis. The chemical energy is then used by plants to make carbohydrates, proteins and fats. We need energy to operate our body, but we cannot use solar energy directly. Instead we get the energy we need from the chemical energy contained in plants or other animals. When we eat food containing carbohydrates, proteins and fats, they are oxidized producing energy, carbon dioxide, water – and heat. This chapter contains a brief discussion of energy, as it generally pertains to our bodies, and how energy relates to weight control.

Energy Conservation

One of the greatest scientific achievements of the nineteenth century was the recognition and statement of the principle of conservation of energy by Julius Robert Von Mayer, in a classic paper written in 1842.. The principle is based on observation of physical phenomenon and states that energy may be converted or transferred but cannot be created or destroyed. Then in 1847, Von Helmholtz, a surgeon in the Prussian army, wrote a brilliant paper applying the principle to the sciences of physiology and chemistry. By the beginning of the twentieth century, the scientific observations of Rubner, and then Atwater and Benedict, had demonstrated the validity of the law of the conservation of energy for the human metabolism.

According to the law of conservation of energy – as related to humans – the energy value of the food eaten (minus the energy lost in waste) must equal the sum of the heat energy leaving the body plus the physical work done by the body. An overwhelming number of scientists today agree that weight change in human beings is linked to their energy balance (or imbalance), and that **weight loss in humans is governed by the law of the conservation of energy**.

Total Energy Requirements

How much energy do you need to maintain your present weight? To answer this question you must understand that an adult's energy requirement consists of three parts: 1) Basal metabolic energy, 2) Activity energy, and 3) Thermic energy. As illustrated in the following figure, the total amount of energy we expend everyday is the sum of the basal energy and the energy expended in physical activity. Our energy source is the food we eat minus waste.

Basal metabolic energy is used to perform the body's involuntary basal processes, such as blood circulation, respiration, glandular activity, contraction of the intestines, body-temperature control, operation of the kidneys, etcetera. All of these functions consume energy. Scientists determine basal energy expenditure, also called basal metabolic rate (BMR), by a carefully controlled test in which measurements are made while a person who hasn't eaten in 14 hours lies quietly and completely relaxed in a comfortably warm room. Results from these tests show that basal metabolic energy is dependent on gender, age, weight and height, and that most people vary within plus and minus ten percent of what is considered normal.

When you reach your mid to late twenties, you slowly start to lose muscle and add fat as part of the natural aging process. But muscle is metabolically active tissue. This means your muscles use calories when they work, as well as when they repair and refuel. Fat, on the other hand, requires very few calories to exist. The conversion of muscle to fat as you age is the reason your basal metabolic rate decreases as you get older. In general, women have lower basal metabolic rates than men because they generally have less muscle than men.

Note that **a safe way to increase your basal metabolic rate is to convert fat to lean body tissue (muscle) by doing strengthening exercises**, such as those described earlier in this eBook

Activity Energy & Activity Levels

As soon as you begin to move about, the physical activity causes your energy output to increase significantly above your basal level. Many experiments have been performed to determine the energy used during various activities. Scientists express the results in terms of calories used per pound of body weight per unit of time. To compute your total daily energy requirement due to physical activity, therefore, would require that you keep a diary of the amount of time spent at each activity for an entire day; your total activity energy for the day would then be calculated by multiplying the amount of time spent at each activity by the caloric value per unit of time for each activity. This approach is fine in a science lab, but in the real world such a detailed determination is impractical.

To overcome this drawback, a number of years ago in an earlier publication this writer devised a more accessible measure of daily physical activity called the Activity-Level method. Essentially, to use the Activity-Level method, you make a judgment as to how active you are. Admittedly, this is the least quantitative topic in this eBook. Nevertheless, it is the most workable in practical, daily living situations. The two most common activity levels are covered in this text:

1) <u>Relatively Inactive During and after Work</u>: This is self-explanatory. It applies to individuals who sit at a desk most of the day and engage in no after-hours exercise.

2) <u>Moderately Active During or After Work</u>: To qualify for this category, you would have to either have a physically strenuous job (such as a construction worker, postal worker delivering mail on foot, etcetera), or engage in some form of regular exercise <u>everyday</u> after work (e.g., taking a brisk three-mile walk, working out in a gym, and so forth).

Once you settle on your Activity Level, you are ready to use the Weight Loss Prediction and Weight Maintenance Calorie tables in the sections that follow.

You Generate Heat When You Eat

In a classic experiment in calorimetry (heat energy measurement), the famous French scientist Lavoisier discovered that the ingestion of food caused an increase in the heat produced by the body. This heat increase is due to the energy required to chew and digest the food and to eliminate the waste. Nutritionists labeled this process the thermic effect of food or specific dynamic action. Note that thermic effect energy was taken into account in deriving the weight control equations used to produce the tables in this eBook.

Yet another factor that influences the amount of energy expended by the body is the ambient or environmental temperature. At low temperatures more heat is lost, but in temperate climates where people are well-clothed and houses are well-heated the effect of ambient temperature is negligible.

The Weight Loss Program

You probably have tried many of the popular diets. I think you will agree that a major shortcoming of these popular quick-weight loss diets is that they lack quantitative information. In addition, many of these fads are neither medically nor scientifically sound. The Weight Control program is different!

How? First, it is the most logical and scientifically reliable weight-loss diet you will ever use. (You will be shown what to do and told why.) Next, the diet is based on the latest science. (You will develop an understanding that will allow you to choose among diet options. You will know numerically what is possible, what will happen and when.) Finally, the Weight Loss Program in this eBook is based on unassailable nutritional practices – no fads here. In short, you will be shown how to construct your own personalized weight loss program as follows:

1) Determine your activity level.
2) Set your weight loss goal and the rate at which you should lose weight.
3) Determine your diet options from the Weight Loss Prediction Tables and choose your caloric intake and duration of your diet.
4) Analyze your eating habits and decide how you will spread your calories, first among the days of the week, and then over the meals of the day.

5) Translate the calorie values into meal types and then actual food portions using a weight loss worksheet.

All of these points and more will be covered later in this chapter. Remember dieting isn't easy. Be assured, however, that if you stay with the program you will lose weight. But before you start to plan your program, you need to understand some fundamental concepts.

When Does Weight Change Occur?

According to the conservation of energy principle, when the energy value of the food consumed minus waste, equals the sum of the basal energy and the energy expended during physical activity, the human body is said to be in energy equilibrium. In this case, that is **when the food energy taken in equals the total energy expended, weight is neither gained nor lost.** When there is an energy imbalance, however, weight is either gained or lost. In general, we can state:

- Weight Gain occurs when your food energy intake is greater than the total energy you expend. In this case your body stores the extra energy as fat.

- Weight Loss occurs when your food energy intake is less than the total energy you expend. In this case your body converts stored fat (and in some cases muscle) into energy.

The measure of energy, whether in the form of food, physical activity, or heat, is the kilocalorie (hereafter simply called the Calorie). As mentioned previously, weight loss occurs when you eat fewer calories than the calories you use in daily living. This difference in calories is referred to as the calorie deficit. How much weight you lose depends on the magnitude of the calorie deficit. In technical terms, **the calorie deficit, or calorie difference, is the driving force for weight change**. (Techies will appreciate that the calorie deficit which is the driving force for weight change is somewhat analogous to a voltage difference which is the driving force for the flow of electricity, and to a temperature difference which is the driving force for the flow of heat.)

What About Counting Carbs?

Every so often a low carbohydrate fad diet becomes popular and its adherents start monitoring the number of carbohydrate grams they consume. You will notice that no special mention of carbohydrates was made in the preceding section concerning weight change. This is because eating too many calories will result in weight gain, whether the calories are from protein, fat, or carbohydrate. In theory it does not matter what foods the calories are from.

Because carbohydrates contain 4 Calories per gram, if you restrict carbohydrates you are indirectly reducing the number of calories you eat, and you will lose weight. But why count carbs when it's calories that are causing the weight loss? In fact, researchers have shown that whether you are trying to lose weight or just maintain your weight, it's calories that count. In theory it does not matter what foods the calories are from – **to lose weight you have to eat fewer calories than you burn.**

Count Weight Watchers' Points?

A recent article in the *Journal of the American Medical Association* reported that people who followed the Weight Watchers Points program for two years only lost an average of six pounds. Despite this, we think Weight Watcher's is a sensible well-balanced weight-loss program, but we do not think their points system is useful.

Their points formula is: Points = (Calories/50) + (Fat grams/12) – (Fiber grams/5). Weight Watchers probably devised this formula to encourage dieters to eat foods that are lower in fat and higher in fiber. A good idea – wrong solution. As discussed earlier, weight loss occurs when your food energy intake is less than the total energy you expend. What dieters need to know is the energy value of a food, and the measure of the energy in food is the calorie – not points. Because the Weight Watchers formula considers fat and fiber, it diminishes the influence of the most important parameter in weight loss, a food's calorie value. In our opinion, Weight Watchers use of points rather than calories is unnecessary, confusing, and counter-productive. **Keep track of what really counts – calories**.

Weight Loss Diets

Sure you want to lose weight but what diet should you choose? Low carb, high protein, low fat? Atkins, Zone, South Beach, Pritikin, or Ornish? What about the grapefruit diet or Sugar Busters? And on and on. Each fad diet that comes along promises to be the true path to weight loss.

In reality you can lose weight on almost any diet. Many of the aforementioned diets don't even mention the word calorie, but when analyzed carefully it's clear that by restricting certain foods these diets are in fact limiting calories. Again, you lose weight when you eat fewer calories than your body burns. It doesn't matter whether the calories are from protein, carbohydrates or fat. Calories are calories.

Low-fat diets gained popularity in the 1990's. And you can lose weight on a low-fat diet provided you also lower your calorie intake. But in recent years, even the strictest fat-limiting advocates have to admit that not all fats are alike. Some fats are bad for you (saturated and trans fats), but others are actually healthy (polyunsaturated and monounsaturated fats) and should be included in any diet – even a weight-loss diet.

Anecdotal evidence and weight loss research indicates that early on you will probably lose weight faster on a low-carb diet. The reason is two-fold. First at the start of any diet there is usually considerable loss of water – and water loss is particularly high for low-carb diets. But the main reason is that when you exclude carbohydrate-rich foods, you have no choice but to eat more fats and protein. Because fats and protein are digested more slowly than carbohydrates, most people don't feel quite as hungry on a low-carb reducing diet. So they eat less – eat fewer calories overall – and lose weight. The problem with low-carb diets is that they are nutritionally unsound and difficult to stay with over the long haul. So what to do?

The Best Weight-Loss Diets

Every good weight-loss diet must have the following three characteristics:
1) A good diet must provide an understanding of weight control as well as the knowledge needed to reduce your weight to the desired level.
2) A good diet must help you remain healthy while you are losing weight.
3) A good diet must lead you to a healthier way of eating and exercising that will help you, in the long term, keep off the weight you have lost.

The weight-loss diet that fits these constraints is the so-called "balanced diet; " i.e., a diet that is not only low calorie but also nutritionally balanced and complies with the Guidelines for Healthy Eating on page 75.

Weight Loss Math

As stated previously, weight loss occurs when your food energy intake is less than the total energy you expend. This difference in calories is referred to as the calorie deficit. How much weight you lose depends on the magnitude of your calorie deficit.

People on any weight-loss diet invariably want to know how much weight they will lose – and how fast. Simple metabolic calculations make a rough estimate possible. Physiologists have long known that to lose one pound requires a deficit of approximately 3,500 Calories. Therefore, if a person's total calorie deficit over time is known, their weight loss over time can be calculated.

As will be evident later, a 30 year-old female office worker, 5' 4" and 175 pounds, expends about 2,500 Calories in day-to-day living. (In other words, if this woman eats about 2,500 Calories per day she will neither gain nor lose weight.) If she goes on a 1,500 Calorie reducing diet, her daily deficit would be 2,500 – 1,500 = 1,000 Calories. In one week her deficit would be 1,000 Calories per day x 7 days = 7,000 Calories, and she should lose 7,000/3,500, or two pounds.

This computation technique, however, is somewhat crude. Primarily because it does not account for a very important scientific fact: **As you lose weight you actually need fewer calories to maintain your lower weight.** As a result, if your calorie intake remains constant over some period of time, your calorie deficit will decrease during your diet and the rate at which you lose weight also will decrease with time.

Weight Loss Prediction Tables

Fortunately, a more precise determination of the rate of weight loss is possible. Scientists have long known that **weight loss is a function of age, sex, height, weight, physical activity, caloric intake and the duration of the diet (or time on the diet)**. This writer related all these variables in a complex, scientifically based, energy-weight-control equation, published in the *American Journal of Clinical Nutrition*,, and subsequently published a set of 60 Weight Loss Prediction tables. In this edition of Weight Loss for Women you will find an abridged set of six Weight Loss Prediction tables (Tables 26 through 31).

Selecting the Correct Table

Your first task is to choose the correct Weight Loss Prediction Table. The six Weight Loss Prediction Tables are organized by age and two activity levels. To repeat, the two most common activity levels covered in this text:

1) <u>Relatively Inactive During and after Work</u>: (Hereafter often just labeled Inactive.) This is self-explanatory. It applies to individuals who sit at a desk most of the day and engage in no after-hours exercise.

2) <u>Moderately Active During or After Work</u>: (Hereafter often just labeled Active.) To qualify for this category, you would have to either have a physically strenuous job (such as a construction worker, postal worker delivering mail on foot, etcetera), or engage in some form of regular exercise <u>everyday</u> after work (e.g., taking a brisk three-mile walk, working out in a gym, and so forth).

Use Table 24 to find the Weight Loss Prediction Table that's right for you. Click on the appropriate Table No.

Age	Activity Level	Table and Page Number.
18 – 35	Relatively inactive	Table 26 page 98
18 – 35	Moderately active	Table 27 page 99
36 – 55	Relatively inactive	Table 28 page 100
36 – 55	Moderately active	Table 29 page 101
56 – 75	Relatively inactive	Table 30 page 102
56 - 75	Moderately active	Table 31 page 103

Table 24: Weight Loss Prediction Tables

Example:: Consider a 42-year-old woman, who is 5' 4" and 160 pounds, has essentially a sedentary job as a computer programmer and spends most of her free time watching TV. How long will it take her to lose 20 pounds?

First she should choose Table 28, labeled "Weight Loss for Relatively Inactive 36 - 55 year olds." Then she would scan the far left of the table and locate her present weight of 160 pounds; from this number she would run a finger horizontally (to the right) until it intersects the vertical column headed by the 20-pound weight loss she desires. The three numbers at the intersection are the time in days to lose 20 pounds, depending on the diet calories consumed. Specifically, to lose 20 pounds our fictional female's diet calorie options are:

- 900 Calories per day for 56 days.
- 1,200 Calories per day for 72 days.
- 1,500 Calories per day for 99 days.

Which alternative should she choose? Health professionals recommend a gradual weight loss of One to two pounds per week. In this case, that would mean her diet should last 10 to 20 weeks or 70 to 140 days, pointing to the 1,200-Calorie diet option.

Better still would be for this woman to increase her activity level by taking a brisk three-mile walk everyday, and qualifying for the moderately active category (Table 17) which would result in the following shorter-duration diet options:

- 900 Calories per day for 48 days.
- 1,200 Calories per day for 59 days.
- 1,500 Calories per day for 76 days.

Hence, by increasing her activity level, she could decrease the time to lose 20 pounds by 14 to 21 percent – depending on the calorie level she chooses.

Weight Loss Prediction for Women
Relatively Inactive 36 - 55

Present Weight	Diet Calories	Weight Loss – lbs							
		5	10	15	20	30	40	50	60
120 lbs.	900	18	37	57					
	1200	25	52	80					
	1500	41	86	138					
130 lbs.	900	17	34	52	71				
	1200	22	46	71	97				
	1500	34	71	112	157				
140 lbs.	900	15	31	48	65	102			
	1200	20	41	63	87	139			
	1500	29	60	94	131	217			
160 lbs.	900	13	27	41	56	87	121	158	
	1200	17	34	53	72	113	158	210	
	1500	23	47	72	99	159	230	316	
180 lbs.	900	12	24	37	50	77	106	137	171
	1200	15	30	45	61	96	133	174	220
	1500	19	38	59	80	127	180	240	311

Numbers in table indicate time in days to lose weight.

Table 25: Portion of Table 28

Please note that the calorie allowance during a weight loss diet need not be the same for every day of the week. It's the average intake over an entire week that counts. For instance, if the woman in the Example selects a 1,500 Calorie diet (which totals 1,500 x 7 = 10,500 Calories for one week), and her eating pattern is such that she knows she will invariably eat more on weekends, she could plan for 1,200 Calories on weekdays and 2,250 on weekends. In effect, she would then be dieting on weekdays and eating "almost normally" on weekends. This eating pattern would amount to (1,200 x 5) + (2,250 x 2) = 10,500 Calories per week, which would result in the same weight loss outcome as if she consumed 1,500 Calories each and every day of the week.

Table 26: Weight Loss - Inactive Women, 18 - 35

Present Weight	Diet Calories	Weight Loss – lbs							
		5	10	15	20	30	40	50	60
120 lbs.	900	16	33	51					
	1200	22	45	70					
	1500	33	69	110					
130 lbs.	900	15	31	47	64				
	1200	20	40	62	85				
	1500	28	59	92	128				
140 lbs.	900	14	28	44	59	93			
	1200	18	37	56	77	122			
	1500	25	49	79	109	179			
160 lbs.	900	12	25	38	52	80	111	144	
	1200	15	31	47	64	101	141	186	
	1500	20	41	62	86	137	195	264	
180 lbs.	900	11	22	34	46	71	97	126	157
	1200	13	27	41	56	87	120	157	197
	1500	17	34	52	71	111	157	207	266
200 lbs.	900	10	20	31	41	4	87	112	139
	1200	12	24	36	49	76	105	136	169
	1500	14	29	45	61	95	132	172	217
220 lbs.	1200	11	22	33	44	68	93	120	149
	1500	13	26	39	53	83	114	148	185
	1800	16	32	49	67	105	147	193	244
240 lbs.	1200	10	20	30	40	62	85	108	134
	1500	11	23	35	48	74	101	130	162
	1800	14	28	43	58	91	126	164	205

Numbers in table indicate time in days to lose weight.

Table 27: Weight Loss - Active Women, 18 - 35

Present Weight	Diet Calories	Weight Loss – lbs							
		5	10	15	20	30	40	50	60
120 lbs.	900	14	29	44					
	1200	18	37	58		Numbers in table			
	1500	25	52	82		indicate time in days			
130 lbs.	900	13	27	41	56	to lose weight.			
	1200	16	33	52	71				
	1500	22	45	70	97				
140 lbs.	900	12	25	38	51	80			
	1200	15	30	47	64	101			
	1500	19	40	62	85	137			
160 lbs.	900	11	22	33	45	69	96	125	
	1200	13	26	40	54	84	118	155	
	1500	16	32	50	68	108	153	205	
180 lbs.	900	9	19	29	40	61	84	109	135
	1200	11	23	34	47	72	100	131	164
	1500	13	27	42	57	89	125	165	210
200 lbs.	900	9	17	26	36	55	75	97	120
	1200	10	20	31	41	64	88	114	142
	1500	12	24	36	49	76	106	138	174
220 lbs.	1200	9	18	28	37	57	79	101	125
	1500	10	21	32	43	67	93	120	150
	1800	12	25	38	52	81	113	148	186
240 lbs.	1200	8	17	25	34	52	71	91	112
	1500	9	19	29	39	60	82	106	132
	1800	11	22	34	46	71	98	127	159

Table 28: Weight Loss - Inactive Women, 36 - 55

Present Weight	Diet Calories	Weight Loss – lbs							
		5	10	15	20	30	40	50	60
120 lbs.	900	18	37	57		Numbers in table indicate time in days to lose weight.			
	1200	25	52	80					
	1500	41	86	138					
130 lbs.	900	17	34	52	71				
	1200	22	46	71	97				
	1500	34	71	112	157				
140 lbs.	900	15	31	48	65	102			
	1200	20	41	63	87	139			
	1500	29	60	94	131	217			
160 lbs.	900	13	27	41	56	87	121	158	
	1200	17	34	53	72	113	158	210	
	1500	23	47	72	99	159	230	316	
180 lbs.	900	12	24	37	50	77	106	137	171
	1200	15	30	45	61	96	133	174	220
	1500	19	38	59	80	127	180	240	311
200 lbs.	900	11	22	33	45	69	94	121	150
	1200	13	26	40	54	83	115	150	187
	1500	16	33	50	68	106	148	195	248
220 lbs.	1200	12	23	36	48	74	102	132	163
	1500	14	29	44	59	92	127	166	208
	1800	18	37	56	77	120	169	223	286
240 lbs.	1200	11	21	32	44	67	92	118	146
	1500	13	25	39	52	81	112	144	180
	1800	16	32	48	66	103	142	186	235

Table 29: Weight Loss - Active Women, 36 - 55

Present Weight	Diet Calories	Weight Loss – lbs							
		5	10	15	20	30	40	50	60
120 lbs.	900	15	32						
	1200	20	42						
	1500	29	61						
130 lbs.	900	14	29	44	60				
	1200	18	37	57	79				
	1500	25	52	81	113				
140 lbs.	900	13	27	41	55	87			
	1200	16	33	52	71	112			
	1500	22	45	70	97	159			
160 lbs.	900	11	23	35	48	75	103	135	
	1200	14	28	43	59	92	129	171	
	1500	18	36	55	76	121	173	235	
180 lbs.	900	10	21	31	42	65	90	117	146
	1200	12	24	37	51	79	109	143	180
	1500	15	30	46	63	99	139	184	236
200 lbs.	900	9	19	28	38	59	80	103	128
	1200	11	22	33	45	69	95	123	154
	1500	13	26	40	54	84	117	153	193
220 lbs.	1200	9	19	30	40	62	84	109	135
	1500	11	23	35	47	73	101	131	164
	1800	14	28	42	58	90	126	165	209
240 lbs.	1200	9	18	27	36	56	76	98	121
	1500	10	20	31	42	65	89	115	143
	1800	12	24	37	50	78	108	140	176

Numbers in table indicate time in days to lose weight.

Table 30: Weight Loss - Inactive Women, 56 - 75

Present Weight	Diet Calories	Weight Loss – lbs							
		5	10	15	20	30	40	50	60
120 lbs.	900	19	40	62					
	1200	28	58	90					
	1500	49	105	170					
130 lbs.	900	18	36	56	76				
	1200	25	51	79	108				
	1500	40	83	132	188				
140 lbs.	900	16	33	51	70	110			
	1200	22	45	70	96	154			
	1500	33	69	109	152	257			
160 lbs.	900	14	29	44	60	93	130	170	
	1200	18	37	57	78	123	174	232	
	1500	25	52	81	112	181	264		
180 lbs.	900	13	26	39	53	82	113	146	183
	1200	16	32	49	66	104	144	189	240
	1500	21	42	65	89	141	201	270	353
200 lbs.	900	11	23	35	47	79	109	141	175
	1200	14	28	43	58	100	139	181	228
	1500	18	36	55	74	135	190	253	326
220 lbs.	1200	12	25	38	51	73	100	129	160
	1500	15	31	47	64	90	124	161	202
	1800	20	41	62	85	117	163	216	275
240 lbs.	1200	11	23	34	46	71	98	126	156
	1500	14	27	42	57	87	121	156	195
	1800	17	35	53	72	113	158	207	262

Numbers in table indicate time in days to lose weight.

Table 31: Weight Loss - Active Women, 56 - 75

Present Weight	Diet Calories	Weight Loss – lbs							
		5	10	15	20	30	40	50	60
120 lbs.	900	16	34	52					
	1200	22	45	71		Numbers in table indicate time in days to lose weight.			
	1500	33	70	112					
130 lbs.	900	15	31	47	64				
	1200	20	40	62	86				
	1500	28	58	92	129				
140 lbs.	900	14	28	43	59	93			
	1200	18	36	56	76	122			
	1500	24	50	78	109	179			
160 lbs.	900	12	24	37	51	79	110	143	
	1200	15	30	46	63	99	139	185	
	1500	19	39	61	83	133	192	262	
180 lbs.	900	11	22	33	45	69	95	124	154
	1200	13	26	40	54	84	117	153	193
	1500	16	32	50	68	107	151	202	260
200 lbs.	900	10	19	30	40	62	85	109	135
	1200	11	23	35	47	73	101	131	164
	1500	14	28	42	58	90	126	165	209
220 lbs.	1200	10	20	31	42	65	89	115	143
	1500	12	24	37	50	78	108	141	176
	1800	15	30	46	62	98	137	180	229
240 lbs.	1200	9	19	28	38	59	80	103	127
	1500	11	22	33	45	69	95	123	153
	1800	13	26	40	54	84	116	152	191

Weight Loss Rate Will Decrease

It is well known that if your caloric intake on a weight-loss diet is constant, your rate of weight loss will decrease with time. In other words, as you lose weight it will get more difficult, or rather it will take a longer time to lose additional weight!

This declining weight loss rate can be understood by considering a 47-year-old woman, who goes on a 1,500-Calorie Diet. She is relatively inactive, 5' 5" and 180 pounds. Referring to **Table 28** (page 100) you will notice that at the start of her 1,500 Calorie diet, when she weighed 180 pounds, it took 38 days for her to lose the first ten pounds. And that the number of days between 10-pound weight loss increments increased as she lost weight. Toward the end of her diet, it took (311-240 = 71) days for her to lose the last ten pounds and reach her goal of 120 pounds! Why does this happen? To understand this phenomenon you have to jump ahead to **Weight Maintenance Calorie Table**. (Table 36 (page 121) the Weight Maintenance Calorie Table lists how many calories you can eat to neither gain nor lose weight.) From Table 36 we find that before she began her diet, she must have been consuming about 2,533 Calories per day to maintain her weight at 180 pounds. At the start of her 1500-Calorie diet, therefore, her deficit was 2,533 − 1,500 = 1,033 Calories per day, and she would have started losing weight at a rate of (1033 x 7/3,500), a little more than two pounds per week. At the end of her diet, the same table shows that at 120 pounds she would have to eat no more than 1,982 Calories per day to neither gain nor lose weight. Her deficit would have been only 1,982 − 1,500 = 482 Calories per day, and her weight lose rate would have dropped to (482 x 7/3,500), or slightly less than one pound per week.

The message is that **if you want to lose weight at a constant rate over time, you must eat slightly less (or exercise harder) as you lose weight.**

Weight Variations Due to Water

When there is a calorie deficit the resulting weight loss is variable in its composition. Fat, water and protein (muscle, bone mass, etcetera) are lost at different rates at different times in the diet. A relatively high percentage of this weight loss is likely to be water, particularly at the start of a diet. For an average person water accounts for about 70 percent of their total body weight. Muscle tissue is approximately 75 percent water, 20 percent protein and five percent mineral. Body fat contains roughly 50 percent water. Because water is a significant component of weight loss, it is essential to understand how the amount of water in your body varies.

First, **realize that your body weight fluctuates two to three pounds daily – whether on a diet or not**. Your weight is lowest before breakfast and highest in the evening before retiring . In addition, the quantity of water in your body also varies from day to day. Over a reasonable time period, however, it can be stated that the amount of fluid leaving your body will equal the amount entering your body by way of food and drink. The water balance of your body is then said to be in equilibrium.

At the start of a diet, there is usually a considerable loss of water, and since one pint of water weighs about one pound, this initial water loss will appear to be a weight loss. But this weight loss is not "real" because only a small quantity of body tissue has been lost. (Many theories have been proposed to explain this phenomenon but none have been scientifically confirmed.) Changes in body hydration, therefore, cause a higher weight loss during the first week or two of a diet than is shown in the Weight Loss Prediction tables. By the following week, however, the body's water balance will again readjust and the total weight loss should more closely follow the values in the tables.

Another cause of weight fluctuation is water retention in women just prior to their menstrual period. This is not uncommon, but for the female dieter this may appear to be a time when weight is not lost. Again, the body's water balance will return to equilibrium the next week, when weight loss should once more closely follow the numbers in the Weight Loss Prediction table. (The Weight Loss Prediction tables show "real" weight loss.)

The Dreaded Weight Loss Plateau

Many dieters complain that after losing some amount of weight, they get stuck; they reach a so-called "plateau," and stop losing weight – at least for some time period. If this happens to you, you may get discouraged and frustrated and wonder what you should do to break through and start losing weight again. Before we address solutions, let's examine the possible causes of a weight loss plateau.

First, you could actually still be losing weight but at such a such low a rate that your weight loss is masked by the natural daily fluctuations in your weight, and your perception is that you have reached a plateau. The low weight loss rate is no doubt due to the much lower calorie deficit associated with your new lower weight – as described in the previous section "Your Weight Loss Rate Will Decreases Over Time." Recall, as you lose weight it gets increasingly harder to lose additional weight. If this is the case, the solution is to increase your calorie deficit by either reducing your caloric intake or increasing your activity level – or both. This done you should once more see a more detectable weight loss each week.

The most probable cause for a real weight loss plateau, however, is that over time you have become careless, either eating slightly more and/or exercising less. Yet another cause could be temporary water retention as discussed in the preceding section. More than likely it is a combination of all of these factors that makes you believe you have stopped losing weight.

If you encounter a weight loss plateau, the first thing to do is sit back and analyze your eating and exercise patterns. Keep a diet diary, honestly listing everything you eat and the associated calories. (Most people underestimate their caloric intake by at least 15 percent.) Add the calories consumed for a week and divide by seven to compute an average daily caloric intake. Then enter the appropriate Weight Maintenance Calorie table at your current weight and activity level and determine your maintenance

calories. (You can find a list of Weight Maintenance Calorie tables here.)
Next, calculate your all-important daily caloric deficit (maintenance calories
minus your daily caloric intake). Then make an estimate of your expected
weekly weight loss by multiplying your daily caloric deficit by seven and
dividing the result by 3,500.

Weight Loss Maxims

Once the parameters involved in weight loss are related in a mathematical
equation, it is possible to state some principles or maxims. (It is also possible
to deduce most of the following truisms by examining the Weight Loss
Prediction tables.)

1) Given two people the same age, gender and activity level, and on the
same reducing diet, **the heavier person will lose weight faster than the
thinner person**. For instance, according to Table 26, on 1,500 Calories, it
would take a 25-year old, 5'-4", 140-pound woman (relatively inactive) 49
days to lose 10 pounds; whereas the same table indicates a 200-pound female
would only take 29 days to lose 10 pounds.

2) Given two people the same age, gender and activity level, and on the
same reducing diet (i.e., consuming the same number of calories), the **taller
person will lose weight at a faster rate**.

3) Given a male and female, the same age, weight, activity level and on the
same reducing diet, **the man will lose weight faster than the woman**. This
is because women most often have less muscle mass and, therefore, lower
basal metabolic rates than men.

4) Given two individuals, the same gender, weight and activity level, **the
younger person will lose weight faster than the older person**. The lesson
is if you are overweight start on a weight loss diet now because it will only
become **more difficult to lose weight as you get older.**

5) It follows that if your **caloric intake is constant over the years you will
slowly gain weight as you age.** This is because you naturally lose muscle
and your basal metabolic rate decreases as you advance in age, and most
people tend not to be as active as they get older.

6) If your **caloric intake on a weight-loss diet is constant, your rate of
weight loss will decrease with time.** Hence, to lose weight at a constant rate
over time, you must eat slightly less (or exercise harder) as you lose weight.

Weight Loss Eating Patterns

Using the nutrition and weight loss information presented to this point, you
should be able to plan a reducing diet suited to your individual likes and
lifestyle. This offers great flexibility, but requires that you take care and use
the **Guidelines for Healthy Eating** (page 75) when choosing foods from all
six-food groups.

After you determine your daily diet calorie allowance from the Weight Loss Prediction Tables, the next step is to decide on a weekly routine, i.e., how you will distribute your calories among the days of the week. As already mentioned your caloric allowance need not be the same for every day of the week. Next apportion your daily caloric allowance among the meals of the day according to your personal eating habits. The following approximate daily calorie distributions are suggestions only. (Feel free, however, to modify this calorie distribution to suit your particular eating routine and lifestyle.)

	900	1,200	1,500
Breakfast	200	200	250
Lunch	250	250	350
Dinner	450	670	780
Snacks	0	80	150

Suggested Daily Calorie Distribution

Set Meals for Calorie Control

Are you concerned about having to count calories? Whether on a reducing diet or trying to maintain your weight, allocating a specific number of calories for each meal makes it unnecessary to keep a running calorie tally for an entire day. Instead, you only need to monitor the number of calories eaten at each meal – and there are ways to keep even this to a minimum by utilizing a concept called "Set Meals" – a strategy not very different than the measured-food-to-eat systems used by diet plans such as Jenny Craig and NutriSystem. Except with the "Set Meals" system you control what you eat.

A Set Meal is a food serving where the ingredients vary - but is almost identical in calorie count and nutritional content day after day. Any meal during the day that is completely under your control is a Set Meal candidate.

For instance, suppose you prepare breakfast at home almost every day. Plan perhaps three set breakfasts. One might be based on cereal and fruit, another on eggs and toast, and so on. Variety is obtained by having more than one choice for a Set Meal, and by eating different kinds of cereal, or fruit, or egg preparations (scrambled, over easy, soft-boiled) – all within the same Set Meal. Once this is done, the number of calories in each of the Set Meal can be easily calculated. Then, try to plan set meals for lunch.

The more Set Meals you have in a day, the less calorie counting. If you have set meals for both breakfast and lunch, then you only have to monitor dinner calories.

Example: Devise a well-balanced, nutritious, weight-loss-eating plan for a 32-year-old woman who wants to start on a 1,500-Calorie diet. A married mother of two, she works full-time as a nurse on the day shift.

First she has to distribute her 1,500 Calories among the meals of the day. Based on her eating habits, as a first pass she decides to allocate approximately 275 Calories for breakfast, 300 for lunch, 650 for dinner and 275 Calories for three snacks. (At this point, these calorie values are tentative and subject to alteration as her eating plan unfolds.)

Next, she has to establish her Set Meals, the meals she has control over, and also account for the foods she likes and dislikes. She certainly has control over breakfast, and she has decided to bring a lunch to the hospital rather than eat in the cafeteria. So she also has control over what she eats for lunch. When she gets home from work, she and her husband prepare dinner together and sometimes they eat out.

For breakfast she likes cereal with skim milk, or eggs and toast. For lunch she prefers things that are quick and easy to prepare like tuna fish, soup, cottage cheese, or cereal (if she hasn't already had cereal for breakfast). She also enjoys a morning and afternoon snack. Now we are ready to layout her meal plan for every day of the week.

Using these facts as input, she establishes the weight loss eating plan broadly outlined in Table 32. Next, she calculates the number of calories in the foods comprising her Set Meals, i.e., her breakfasts and lunches and snacks. The details behind Table 32 are in a spreadsheet (not shown).

	Mon	Tues	Weds	Thurs	Fri	Sat	Sun
Breakfast	Cereal (M)	Toast	Egg	Cereal (M)	Egg	Cereal (M)	Egg
Snack	Fruit	Yogurt & Fruit	Yogurt & Fruit	Fruit	Yogurt & Fruit	Fruit	Yogurt & Fruit
Lunch	Soup	Cereal (S)	Cereal (S)	Tuna	Cereal (S)	Tuna	Cereal (S)
Snack	Nuts & Seeds	Nuts & Seeds	Nuts & Seeds	Nuts & Seeds	Nuts & Seeds	Nuts & Seeds	Nuts & Seeds
Calories	730	805	680	730	730	850	680

Table 32: Weight Loss Eating Plan

For breakfast, "Cereal (M)" consists of a healthy cereal (such as Oat Meal, Wheatena, Farina, Shredded Wheat, Cheerios, Wheat Chex, Wheaties, and some Kashi cereals) with skim milk and topped with a half a banana or other fruit. "Cereal (Y)" substitutes non-fat yogurt for skim milk. In addition, four ounces of fruit juice are part of every breakfast.

For lunch, acceptable soups include tomato, vegetable, pea, actually any soup where a serving is 125 Calories or less. Any low-calorie salad dressing (about 25 Calories per tablespoon) can be used. Remember to use tuna packed in water rather than oil. Worth noting is that every effort was made to nutritionally balance the meals in a given day. For example, either milk, yogurt or cottage cheese are present every day.

Overall variety is achieved by having different brands of cereal, different kinds of fruit, several types of nuts and seeds, different kinds of soup, and eggs prepared in various ways. To make sure she is getting the proper amount of nutrients every day, for dinner she plans to have at least two other vegetable servings, a starch (potato or brown rice), and a small serving of fish, poultry, lean meat, or a plant protein. Her evening snack (dessert) depends on the number of calories she has remaining after dinner. Dessert could be a small glass of skim milk and yes a cookie, or a low-calorie pudding, etcetera. Coffee or tea (with skim milk and an artificial sweetener if desired) can be served at any meal or as part of a snack.

From Table 32 we notice that her calorie total for breakfast, lunch and snacks is not the same for every day of the week. Because it is impractical to assign a different dinner calorie target for every day of the week, we average the daily totals for breakfast, lunch and snacks (as shown in the worksheet), and use the average value to calculate her allowable dinner calories. Table 32 indicates that for dinner (and any evening snack) she is allowed a total of 756 Calories (1500 Calories minus the calories she has already eaten for breakfast, lunch and day-time snacks).

This dinner calorie total should be relatively easy to stay within provided she eats well-balanced meals with portion sizes consistent with her 756 Calorie limit. To understand what "reasonable" portion sizes should look like for a 756-Calorie meal, at first she will probably have to count calories at dinner. After a few weeks of counting dinner calories, however, she should be able to judge what is and what is not an acceptable portion size for the different foods on her plate – and then proceed without actually counting calories.

Using this Set Meal technique, she only has to judge or estimate her dinner calories to assure that she is close to her diet calorie allowance on a weekly basis. If you are uneasy about devising your own weight loss eating plan, either use the pre-planned diets in the next section, or seek the professional advice of a registered dietitian. Registered dietitians translate the science of nutrition into everyday information about food, and are trained to assist people with their individual diets and meal plans. Go online to find a registered dietitian in your area.

Finally, how should she manage the inevitable, i.e., when she has to attend a business luncheon, or an all-day business meeting, or she goes on a vacation? In other words, how should she handle those days when she just can't follow her weight loss eating plan? See page 113.

Pre-Planned Diets

Despite all the information that has been provided here, if you would rather not go through the trouble of planning a personal diet eating routine, use one of the pre-planned 900, 1,200, or 1,500 Calorie eating patterns shown in Tables 33 to 35. The diets are recommended because they adhere to the U.S. Department of Agriculture Dietary Guidelines and are nutritionally sound.

900-Calorie Diet

Breakfast A	Breakfast B	Breakfast C
½ cup fruit or juice	½ cup fruit or juice	½ cup fruit or juice
1 oz. (30 g) cereal	1 egg cooked w/o fat	1 oz. (30 g) cereal
1 cup skim milk	1 slice dry toast	6 oz fat-free yogurt
Coffee or tea	Coffee or tea	Coffee or tea
Lunch A	**Lunch B**	**Lunch C**
1 cup fat-free cottage	2 oz. lean meat	3 oz. fish
1 cup vegetables	1 cup vegetables	1 cup vegetables
Coffee or tea	1 slice bread	1 slice bread
	Coffee or tea	Coffee or tea
Dinner A	**Dinner B**	**Dinner C**
2 oz. Chicken	3 oz. fish	3 oz. Chicken
Green salad + dressing	Green salad + dressing	Green salad + dressing
1 slice bread	6 oz fat-free yogurt	1 slice bread
1 cup fruit	Coffee or tea	1 cup fruit
Coffee or tea		Water
905 Cal	**930 Cal**	**930 Cal**

Table 33: 900-Calorie Menus

In most cases, a 900-Calorie diet should be used only under a physician's supervision. Note that two unsweetened gelatin deserts may also be eaten every day at meals or as a snack.

1,200-Calorie Diet

Breakfast A	**Breakfast B**	**Breakfast C**
½ cup fruit or juice	½ cup fruit or juice	½ cup fruit or juice
1 oz. (30 g) cereal	1 egg cooked w/o fat	1 oz. (30 g) cereal
1 cup skim milk	1 slice dry toast	6 oz fat-free yogurt
Coffee or tea	Coffee or tea	Coffee or tea
Lunch A	**Lunch B**	**Lunch C**
1 cup fat-free cottage	2 oz. lean meat	4 oz. fish
1 cup vegetables	1 cup vegetables	1 cup vegetables
Coffee or tea	1 slice bread	1 slice bread
	Coffee or tea	Coffee or tea
Dinner A	**Dinner B**	**Dinner C**
3½ oz. lean meat	4 oz. fish	4 oz. chicken
Green salad + dressing	Green salad + dressing	Green salad + dressing
1 cup vegetables	1 cup vegetables	1 medium potato
1 slice bread	1 slice bread	1 cup fruit
1 cup fruit	1 cup fruit	Coffee or tea
Coffee or tea	Coffee or tea	
1110 Cal	**1120 Cal**	**1125 Cal**

Table 34: 1,200-Calorie Menus

Elective Calorie Budget: In addition to the above, 80 Calories may be used as desired for a snack - such as ½ cup non-fat ice cream, or for one tsp peanut butter to spread on a slice of bread, etc. Further, two unsweetened gelatin deserts may also be eaten every day at meals or as a snack.

1,500-Calorie Diet

Breakfast A	Breakfast B	Breakfast C
½ cup fruit or juice	½ cup fruit or juice	½ cup fruit or juice
1 oz. (30 g) cereal	1 egg cooked w/o fat	1 oz. (30 g) cereal
1 cup skim milk	2 slices dry toast	6 oz fat-free yogurt
1 slice plain toast	Coffee or tea	1 slice plain toast
Coffee or tea		Coffee or tea
Lunch A	**Lunch B**	**Lunch C**
1 cup fat-free cottage	2 oz. lean meat	4 oz. fish
1 cup vegetables	1 cup vegetables	1 cup vegetables
1 slice bread	1 slice bread	1 slice bread
1 cup fruit	6 oz fat-free yogurt	Coffee or tea
Coffee or tea	Coffee or tea	
Dinner A	**Dinner B**	**Dinner C**
3½ oz. lean meat	5 oz. fish	5 oz. chicken
Green salad + dressing	Green salad + dressing	Green salad + dressing
1 cup vegetables	1 cup rice	1 medium potato
1 slice bread	1 cup vegetables	1 cup vegetables
1 cup fruit	1 cup fruit	1 cup fruit
Coffee or tea	Coffee or tea	Coffee or tea
1365 Cal	**1370 Cal**	**1340 Cal**

Table 35: 1,500-Calorie Menus

Elective Calorie Budget: In addition to the above, 140 Calories may be used as desired for a snack - such as ¾ cup low-fat ice cream, or for one tsp peanut butter to spread on a slice of bread, etcetera. Further, two unsweetened gelatin deserts may also be eaten every day at meals or as a snack.

Notice that Tables 33 through 35 contain no recipes. For instance, the 1,200 Calorie Balanced Diet shown in Table 34 specifies ½ cup of vegetables, but does not identify the kind of vegetables and gives no advice regarding how the vegetables should be prepared. This is because Tables 33 to 35 are general diet guidelines around which more specific meals and recipes can be planned to suit individual preferences and taste. Admittedly, the tables reflect typical American eating patterns but are easily modified to accommodate the tastes and traditions of people from other countries.

Again, if you are not sure you can devise your own weight loss eating plan, or the pre-planned diets in the next section are not to your liking, seek the professional help of a registered dietitian.

Pre-Planned Diets Notes

The following notes apply to the 900, 1,200 and 1,500 diets shown in Tables 33 to 35

1) Cereal should be whole grain and preferably unsweetened. At the top of the list are Old-fashioned Oat Meal, Wheatena and Shredded Wheat. Among other reasonably healthy choices are Cheerios, Wheat Chex, Wheaties some Kashi cereals and Farina.

2) Bread may be either plain or toasted whole wheat, whole rye or pumpernickel. If desired, bread may be sprayed with a zero-calorie butter substitute.

3) Meat should be lean cuts with all visible fat trimmed. Poultry should be limited to chicken or turkey breasts (white meat and skinless).

4) An unlimited amount of green salad may be eaten, but the salad dressing should contain no more than 1 tbsp of vegetable oil (olive, canola, sunflower, safflower etcetera).

5) Potato should be baked or boiled and (if desired) served with a tbsp of non-fat sour cream, or sprayed with a zero-calorie butter substitute. Where rice is specified, brown or wild rice is recommended.

6) Use freely as desired: clear unsweetened coffee, clear unsweetened tea, water (with a squeeze of lemon section if desired), seltzer water, and diet soda.

7) Use freely as desired: clear soups w/o fat, bouillon, and seasonings such as mustard, cinnamon, dill, herbs, red and black pepper, curry, vinegar, lemon juice and sections, and dill and sour pickles.

Helpful Diet Strategies

Everyone needs strategies to help stay on the right-diet track. Here are a few time-tested dieting techniques that work. (All are explained in the sections that follow.)

1) Exchange equivalent foods for variety and prevent boredom.

2) To avoid "hidden calories," prepare simple foods cooked in an uncomplicated manner.

3) Get a good cookbook and a calorie reference.

4) Learn to estimate portion sizes.

5) Use Set Meals to make calorie control easy.

6) Handle occasional overeating by compensating.

7) Keep log of what you eat.

8) Use technology to monitor the calories you eat.

9) If it suits your lifestyle, follow a weekly rather a daily calorie allowance.
10) Handle special situations by temporarily going on weight maintenance.
11) Check your progress by graphing your weight loss.
Again all are discussed in some detail in the sections that follow. Choose the strategy (or strategies) that are right for you.

Exchanging Foods

To prevent a diet from becoming monotonous, after a few weeks try exchanging or substituting foods – a technique used by dieticians. Exchanging a food listed in a diet for another food with approximately equal caloric value and nutritional content is the foundation of a successful long-term diet. Substitution possibilities are almost endless but have to be done carefully.

The easiest substitutions are those within the same food group, such as exchanging one vegetable variety for another, or a glass of milk for a cup of yogurt.   More sophisticated exchanges cross food groups, for instance replacing four ounces of lean meat with a tablespoon of peanut butter spread on a piece of whole wheat bread. Both foods are complete protein and both contain about 170 Calories.

Simple is Better

When on a diet simple is better. Why? Because simple, uncomplicated meals will usually contain fewer "hidden calories" than more elaborate dishes. For example, straightforward broiled fish with micro-waved vegetables makes a nutritious, quick, low-calorie dinner – with no "hidden calories." To add interest to foods without adding calories, season with spices and condiments.

Get a Good Cookbook & Calorie Ref

Acquire a good low-calorie cookbook. Be sure the recipes cover breakfast, lunch and dinner, and all the recipes contain nutritional information, especially the number of calories per serving. In addition, **obtain a comprehensive food calorie guide** such as the excellent U.S. D. A. Home and Garden Bulletin No. 72: "Nutritive Value of Foods," which is online and can be downloaded at no cost.

Estimating Portion Sizes

Whatever calorie counting scheme you use, another dilemma for dieters is judging portion size. It makes no sense to worry about whether to apportion 70 or 80 Calories per ounce for a cut of lean meat if you have no idea whether the portion you are planning to eat weighs four or ten ounces. You must learn to estimate portion sizes with reasonable accuracy. The best way to do this is to start by weighing and measuring the food you eat. After about a week or two, your eye should be adjusted to what four ounces of meat or six ounces of fish look like, and you can then discontinue weighing.

Incidentally, judging the weight of meat or poultry will be one of the most important parts of your diet. As a guide, four ounces of meat or poultry is about the standard size of a slice of bread 4 x 4 x ¼ inch. And calorie tables always refer to meat that has been cooked and trimmed of visible fat and bone.

How to Handle Overeating

It's a fact of life that no matter how determined you are to abide by your daily calorie goal, life has a way of interfering. In real life, you probably will not be able to eat the same number of calories day after day. Maybe it's your social life that interferes. Maybe you have to attend a wedding reception. Maybe an unexpected occasion arises where you know you're going to go over your daily calorie allowance. What should you do?

The way to handle the inevitable overeating is by compensating. You compensate by estimating how far you have strayed from your weight-loss diet and then make amends at the next opportunity (usually the next meal or two) – by eating less.

For instance, let's say you have to attend a business luncheon. Further, assume the meal has been pre-ordered so you have no choice but to eat what's served. At some point toward the end of the meal, make a mental estimate of the number of calories you have eaten. Suppose, even though you tried to be careful, your estimate is about 850 Calories. If your normal Set Lunch is 450 Calories, you know you have over done it by approximately 400 Calories. That night at dinner you decide to have water instead of wine, to forgo your evening snack and to take a half hour after-dinner walk. By doing this, before the end of the day, you will have compensated for the extra 400 Calories you ate at lunch.

Eating in Restaurants: To eat as few calories as possible, during your weight-loss diet adhere to the following restaurant guidelines. First, for an appetizer order fruit juice or melon. For your main course order broiled fish, poultry or a lean cut of meat cooked as plainly as possible (no butter, stuffing, gravy). Order steamed vegetables and maybe a baked potato. Have your salad with the dressing on the side. Finally, ask for fruit for dessert – or have just coffee or tea.

Keep a Log of What You Eat

Behavior research indicates that dieters who keep a record of what they eat generally have more successful outcomes. How should you go about this? Keep a food log. One day of a sample Daily Food Log is shown in Table 36.

The dieter's goal was 1,200 Calories. The actual total for the day was 1,240 Calories. Not bad!

You can keep your daily food log in a small notebook, a daily planner, a laptop, or Smart Phone, whatever works best for you. As shown, you should record the date, meal, food eaten, amount, calorie estimate, total calories for the day and any comments. To approximate the weight of a portion or serving use either a small scale or visually estimate the weight by employing rules of thumb, such as four ounces of meat or fish is about the size of a deck of cards, and one and one-half ounces of cheese is similar in size to a pair of dice. Once you know the weight, use either **Table 23** (page 83), "Calorie Rank (per ounce) of Common Foods," or a more comprehensive calorie reference to determine the calories in a particular portion.

Diet Tip: The secret to a healthy weight loss diet is to make every calorie count in terms of your nutritional needs.

Meal	Food	Amount	Calories
Breakfast Monday 07/12	Juice	half cup	55
	Cereal	cup	110
	Skim milk	half cup	40
	Black coffee		0
Snack	Tea		0
Lunch	Cottage cheese	cup	160
	Broccoli	half cup	25
	Bread	slice	75
Snack	Tea & cracker		60
Dinner	Salmon	4 oz	200
	Baked potato	medium	100
	Salad + oil	1 tbsp	140
	Mixed veggies	half cup	45
	Bread	slice	75
	Apple	medium	75
	Skim milk	cup	80
		Total	1240

Table 36 Daily Food Log

Handling Special Situations

Suppose you are in the middle of your diet and you have to travel overseas for a few weeks, or you have to leave on a planned three-week family vacation. In both circumstances you know you will never be able to resist the food and stay on your diet. What to do?

One solution is to go off your diet – temporarily. Essentially go on weight maintenance and try to at least return from your trip or vacation without having gained any weight. (Weight Maintenance is covered in the next chapter where you will learn how many calories you can eat to neither gain nor lose weight.) When you get back, you can pick up where you left off – back on your diet and resume your weight loss.

Plot Your Weight Loss

Another technique to help you track your weight loss progress, is to graphically compare your actual weight loss to your expected weight loss from the Weight Loss Prediction table that applies to you. If you're computer savvy you can plot your weight loss on your computer using a graphical software package. Otherwise, just use ordinary graph paper. Either way proceed as follows.

First, from the Weight Loss Prediction Table appropriate for your gender, age, and activity level, choose your diet calorie level. Next, using the data in the table, plot your predicted weight loss versus time on the diet. Draw a solid line through the data points. This is your baseline against which you will compare your actual weight loss. Weigh in at the start of your diet. Then, once a week, weigh yourself first thing in the morning and plot the value. If your weight loss is less than the predicted values, most likely you are either 1) cheating (eating more than your diet calorie allowance), or you're not as active as you think, as the weight loss prediction table you're using requires – or both.

Can You Target Weight Loss?

As you gain weight, a host of factors, the most important of which are genetics, gender, and age, determine where on your body you will put down fat. Let's say you have a particular area that's collected a lot of fat and it's bothering you – maybe it's around your abdomen (belly fat), your thighs or under your chin. Is there anything you can do to eliminate or just reduce the amount of fat in a particular annoying area? **The short answer is no**, but read on.

Losing Belly Fat

The truth of the matter is that your body decides where to put fat on and where to remove it, a system that is largely determined by your genetics. Your body distributes fat based on tactics developed over the eons.

Fat is stored in your abdomen, hips or buttocks because it takes less energy to carry fat accumulated in your midsection than other areas of your body. Keep in mind fat storage is a survival strategy, so your body tends to maximize energy efficiency in the formation, storage and use of body fat. Then, from an anthropological viewpoint, the location of body fat has reproductive implications. In women, fat is stored in the hips, buttocks and breasts to create a more attractive body in order to attract a potential mate. Lastly, your body amasses fat where you have put down fat cells when you were young.

Getting rid of abdominal fat has, undoubtedly, as great a level of misunderstanding as any weight loss subject. The major fallacy is that you can get rid of abdominal fat by working your abdominal muscles. This is based on the incorrect belief that fat is eliminated from a part of your body if you engage the muscles underneath that layer of fat. No such luck.

Last On First Off

This **general weight-change rule (based on observation) is "last on first off."** Assume as you gained weight, the first place you noticed it was on your thighs, next your buttocks, then your face. As you lose weight, it generally will come off in the reverse order, first from your face, then your rear and finally your thighs. And there is not much you can do about that. The truth is there is no food, no exercise, no magic belt, and no pill that will cause your body to lose fat in one place rather than another.

For women, this means the last place you're likely to lose fat is on your hips and buttocks. You may have already observed this phenomenon if you've ever been on a diet, or if you've lost weight but couldn't seem to lose that last bit of "stubborn" body fat.

For men, abdominal fat is probably the last fat that will disappear from your body. In the most likely progression, first you will lose fat from your face and extremities, such as your arms and legs, then from your upper torso, your chest, upper thighs and buttocks, and finally the fat stored in your abdomen. And science has not devised a technique to alter this fat reduction pattern.

So if you are really serious about getting rid of that abdominal fat, you're going to have to take a whole-body approach – and get used to the idea that belly fat is likely to be the last fat to go. This isn't what you want to hear, but it's the truth. To reduce body fat, you need to start consuming fewer calories than you expend on a daily basis. In other words, you need a calorie deficit. In time, your body will start converting fat into useable energy, and by doing so, fat stores will begin to disappear all across your body. But fat won't just magically vanish from one targeted place.

If you follow a healthy weight-loss diet combined with aerobic exercise and strength training, you will lose weight and eventually that weight loss will eliminate or reduce your particular problem area. In summary, despite what you may have read, there is no diet regimen or exercise routine that can "target" a particular area of your body. Just be patient and as you lose weight that problem area will eventually disappear.

Words of Caution

A reducing diet is best supervised by a physician. This is especially true when a great deal of weight needs to be lost, or if you have an ailment or a history of medical problems. The Weight Loss Prediction tables cover a wide range of possibilities. And while the values in the tables are theoretically attainable, they are not necessarily recommended for everyone. In some cases the wide ranges were computed and included for completeness.

Most physicians recommend that weight loss should be limited to no more than one to two pounds per week, except for very large individuals, or if the total amount of weight to be lost is very small. In these cases, an acceptable weight loss rate may be as high as three pounds per week. And many nutritionists feel that weight-loss diets should not have food intakes below 900 to 1200 Calories. This is because it is difficult to obtain the proper amount of essential nutrients below these levels.

Don't Give Up!

Finally, realize that, in all likelihood, the road to your weight loss goal will not be an easy one. You didn't gain all that extra weight last week, did you? No, of course not. You probably accumulated the extra weight over the course of several years. No doubt it was a slow, gradual change that occurred because your daily caloric intake during that time exceeded your daily caloric expenditure by some small amount. The point is that small but permanent changes in your diet can put you back on track and create the permanent weight loss you desire.

Don't get frazzled if you have a few setbacks along the way. Many dieters think that if they have a weekend or even a week where they eat more than they should, they might as well give up. Not true. Many successful dieters have lots of bad days. But they don't expect to be perfect. When you hit a bump in the road, simply take a break, relax, and re-start your diet. Successful dieters know that losing weight is a journey – with good days and some bad days – all are expected as they proceed along the road toward their weight loss goal.

WEIGHT MAINTENANCE

Most diet books either ignore or glance over weight maintenance. So the dieter who has somehow lost weight is left without any post-dieting guidelines regarding how to maintain their new lower weight. This purpose of this chapter is to help you maintain your hard earned weight loss.

The Weight Maintenance Program

In this chapter you will be introduced to the information you need to understand to successfully maintain your new weight level. You will learn how to apply the following to establish your own personalized a weight maintenance plan:

1) Use the Weight Maintenance Calorie Tables, to determine how many calories per day you may eat without gaining or losing a significant amount of weight.

2) Analyze your eating habits and decide how you will spread your maintenance calories, first among the days of the week, and then over the meals of an individual day.

3) Translate the calorie values into meal types and then actual food portions using a weight maintenance worksheet.

Again, each of these points will be elaborated on later in this chapter.

Why Do People Regain Weight?

Within five years, more than 90 percent of all dieters regain every pound they have lost. Why? In most cases it's because after losing weight most people eventually revert to their pre-diet eating and exercising habits, and this inevitably leads to their regaining the weight they lost – and often more. The fact is the less you weigh, the less you need to eat to sustain your lower weight. The quantity of food energy required to <u>maintain</u> a particular weight is again a function of sex, age, height, weight and activity level, as is clearly shown in Weight Maintenance Calorie Tables that follow.

<u>Example</u>: Let's consider a 53-year-old relatively inactive woman who weighed 200 pounds at the start of her reducing diet. After losing 50 pounds, she weighed 150 pounds.   Determine her weight maintenance calories before and after she lost weight.

From Table 37 find that before she started her diet, when she weighed 200 pounds, her weight maintenance level was 2,705 Calories, meaning she must have been eating about 2,705 Calories of food per day. After her diet, the same table shows that in order to maintain her lower weight of 150 pounds she must restrict her food intake in the future to 2,265 Calories per day. On average, then, to neither gain nor lose weight at 150 pounds she must consume about 440 Calories per day less than she did when she weighed 200 pounds.

This person could help her cause by engaging in some form of exercise everyday. For example, if she walked 45 minutes every day at moderate 3.5 mph pace (covering a distance of slightly more than 2½ miles), she could eat an additional (297 − 88) x 45 / 60 = 157 Calories per day without gaining weight. (See **Table 8** (page 23)"Calories Burned for Different Activities.)

Weight Maintenance Calories

Weight (lbs)	Age: 18-35 years		Age: 36-55 years		Age: 56-75 years	
	Inactive	Active	Inactive	Active	Inactive	Active
100	1885	2042	1782	1939	1708	1865
105	1938	2103	1833	1998	1758	1923
110	1991	2164	1883	2056	1806	1979
115	2042	2223	1933	2114	1855	2036
120	2093	2282	1982	2171	1902	2091
125	2144	2340	2031	2227	1949	2146
130	2194	2398	2079	2283	1996	2200
135	2243	2455	2126	2338	2042	2254
140	2291	2512	2173	2393	2088	2308
145	2340	2568	2219	2447	2133	2361
150	2387	2623	2265	2501	2177	2413
160	2481	2733	2356	2608	2266	2517
170	2574	2841	2445	2713	2352	2620
180	2665	2948	2533	2816	2438	2721
190	2754	3053	2619	2918	2522	2821
200	2843	3157	2705	3019	2605	2920
210	2930	3260	2789	3119	2688	3018
220	3016	3362	2872	3218	2769	3115
230	3101	3463	2955	3316	2849	3211
240	3185	3563	3036	3414	2929	3306
250	3269	3662	3117	3510	3008	3401

Table 37: Weight Maintenance Calories

Weight – a Life-Long Struggle

A study, published in the Annals of Internal Medicine, that followed 4,000 people for three decades suggests that in the long term, 90 percent of men and 70 percent of women will become overweight (with a BMI ≥ 25). Interestingly, half of the men and women in the study, who had made it well into adulthood without a weight problem, ultimately also became overweight and a third became obese (with a BMI ≥ 30). The point being that you can never become complacent. **You must continually watch your weight because we are all at risk of becoming overweight.**

When you reach your mid to late twenties, you slowly start to lose muscle and add fat as part of the natural aging process. But muscle is metabolically active tissue. This means your muscles use calories when they work, as well as when they repair and refuel. Fat, on the other hand, requires very few calories to exist. This is one of the reasons you need fewer calories to remain at the same weight as you get older.

In weight maintenance, it is the number of calories you eat over the long term that is important. As an illustration, the weight maintenance value of 2,297 Calories per day for the 53-year-old woman in the previous example amounts to about 838,000 Calories in a single year. Now realize that an annual error of only two percent of this total (that is roughly 16,800 Calories per year, or 46 Calories per day) would result in a weight gain of almost five pounds in one year, and the importance of knowing and adhering to your personal weight maintenance calorie value becomes apparent. In brief, **to control your weight it is the number of calories eaten over the long term that matters**.

Obviously, it would be impossible for the woman in the example to eat exactly 2,297 Calories day after day . Errors are inevitable and experience has shown that when people err they do so on the high side. They consume more calories than their maintenance value, rarely less. To allow for occasional overeating or days when you can't get in some exercise, it is recommended that you plan to eat about seven percent below the calorie values in the weight maintenance tables. For the female in the previous example, that would result in about 2,140 Calories per day rather than the 2,297 Calories shown in the weight maintenance calorie table – leaving her room for an occasional calorie splurge, or a missed exercise session.

Planning Maintenance Eating

Weight maintenance begins once you are at your "best weight," or achieve a weight that feels right for you. Weight maintenance is in fact more difficult than being on a weight-loss diet. Why? Chiefly because maintenance requires a life-long commitment, a commitment to a new life style where you eat balanced, nutritious meals that are within your maintenance calorie allowance.

Any motivational speech made at this point isn't going to be much help five and ten years down the road – when I trust you will still be in maintenance mode. Understand that if you really want to keep off the weight you have lost you will have to practice a good deal of self-discipline for a long time. Even the well motivated, however, need a good plan to succeed. The following approach (which is very similar to that discussed in the preceding "Planning Weight Loss Eating Patterns") is recommended:

1) Use the Weight Maintenance Calorie table that applies to you to determine your daily weight-maintenance calorie allowance.

2) Then decide on a weekly routine, i.e., how your calorie allowance is to be distributed among the days of the week. (As stated previously our caloric intake need not be the same for every day of the week.)

3) Next allocate the daily caloric allowance among the meals of the day according to your eating habits.

Obviously, a detailed meal plan for every possible calorie level cannot be included here, but given the information that is covered in Appendix A: Nutrition, it should be possible to plan eating patterns you can live with for any weight maintenance calorie allowance. (See the example that follows immediately). Granted this will take some work but in the long run it will be time well spent.

Example: Devise a weight maintenance eating plan for a 58-year-old woman who, after losing 20 pounds, weighs 180 pounds. She describes her activity level as relatively inactive. An engineering consultant, she works out of an office in her home.

First, from Table 37, she finds her maintenance calorie level is approximately 2,533 Calories per day.) To determine how many calories per day she should plan to consume, she deducts a safety factor of seven percent from 2,533 to allow for occasional overeating (or under-exercising). The result is about 2,350 Calories per day – the number of maintenance calories she plans to eat on most days. Then, she has to establish the meals she has control over (these will be her Set Meals), and also account for the foods she likes and dislikes. Because on most days she is home all day, she has control over every meal except dinner. (When her husband gets home from work, they prepare dinner together or sometimes go out to eat.)

For breakfast the woman in the example likes cereal (with skim or soy milk) or eggs, and for lunch she prefers a tuna sandwich, soup or cereal (if she hasn't already had cereal for breakfast). She also wants to allow for a morning and afternoon snack. Now she is ready to layout her meal plan for every day of the week. The resulting maintenance eating plan is broadly outlined in Table 38

Next, she calculates the number of calories in the foods comprising her Set Meals, i.e., her breakfasts, lunches and snacks. The details behind Table 38 are not shown here (because of size limitations).

	Mon	Tues	Weds	Thurs	Fri	Sat	Sun
Breakfast	Cereal (M)	Toast	Egg	Cereal (M)	Egg	Cereal (M)	Egg
Snack	Fruit	Yogurt & Fruit	Yogurt & Fruit	Fruit	Yogurt & Fruit	Fruit	Yogurt & Fruit
Lunch	Soup	Cereal (S)	Cereal (S)	Tuna	Cereal (S)	Tuna	Cereal (S)
Snack	Nuts & Seeds	Nuts & Seeds	Nuts & Seeds	Nuts & Seeds	Nuts & Seeds	Nuts & Seeds	Nuts & Seeds
Calories	1,175	955	1,075	1,100	1,075	1,100	1,075

Table 38: Maintenance Eating Plan

As shown in Table 38, Cereal (M) indicates a cereal mix with skim milk, and that four ounces of juice are included with every breakfast choice. Worth noting is that every effort was made to balance the meals in a given day.

To assure she is getting an adequate amount of nutrients every day, for dinner she always intends to have a large salad, at least two other vegetable servings, a starch (potato or brown rice), and a small serving of fish, poultry, lean meat, or a plant protein. Her evening snack (dessert) frequently includes a glass of skim milk and yes a few cookies. (Nobody is perfect!)

Overall variety is achieved by having different brands of cereal, different kinds of fruit, several types of nuts and seeds, different soup, and eggs prepared in various ways. In addition, to introduce even more variety, every few months she will revisit her plan and make some adjustments to her Set Meals by adding and subtracting foods.

For dinner, her calorie allowance is her maintenance calories minus the calories she has already eaten for breakfast, lunch and snacks Note that her calorie total for breakfast, lunch and snacks is not the same for every day of the week. This is not unexpected. Because it is unrealistic to assign a different dinner calorie target for every day of the week, she averages the daily totals for breakfast, lunch and snacks (as shown in the worksheet), and uses the average value to calculate his allowable calories for dinner. She determines that she can eat 1,000 Calories for dinner. This dinner calorie total should satisfy the appetite of the woman in the example and should be easy to stay within provided she eats well-balanced meals with "reasonable" portion sizes. To understand what "reasonable" portion sizes should look like for a 1,000-Calorie meal, at first she will probably have to count calories at dinner. After a few weeks of counting dinner calories, however, she should be able to judge what is and what is not an acceptable portion size for the different foods on her plate – without actually counting calories.

Using the Set Meal technique, she only has to judge or estimate her dinner calories to assure that she is close to her maintenance calories on a weekly basis. This plan should make it easier for her to control what she eats and maintain her new lower weight over the long haul. Once again, if you are not sure you can devise your own weight maintenance eating plan, seek the professional advice of a registered dietitian.

Finally, how should she manage the inevitable, i.e., when she has to attend a business luncheon, or an all-day business meeting, or she goes on a vacation? In other words, how should she handle those days when he just can't follow her weight maintenance eating plan? Briefly, she knows her maintenance eating pattern is approximately 400 Calories for breakfast, 500 Calories for lunch, 200 Calories for snacks, 1,000 Calories for dinner and 250 Calories for dessert. And if she has been following this pattern for some time, she should be able to recognize the kinds of food and the amounts (portion sizes) that make up the calories she is allowed at each meal. Then with the added understanding of how to estimate the calorie content of various foods (see page 84), she should be able to eat meals that approximate the calorie content of her weight maintenance eating plan. Lastly, if this approach does not work for her, she should realize that a day or two off her maintenance eating regimen is not the end of the world.

Mini Diets Maintain Weight Loss

Many people go through life maintaining their weight without thinking about how much they eat or exercise. When they occasionally eat a bigger meal, they seem to automatically eat less at the next meal or they exercise more, or they do both. If for some reason they expend more energy, they instinctively eat more. These people are able to maintain an almost constant weight without any effort. For most of us, however, weight control is more difficult, and we must be vigilant. For us weight control is a relentless life-long challenge.

When on a weight-loss diet, check and record your progress by weighing yourself at the same time two or three days per week. Once you are in weight maintenance mode, i.e., you have reached your desired weight level, weigh in about once a week. Small, natural weight fluctuations can be ignored, but action is called for if you experience a "noteworthy" increase in weight. What is a noteworthy weight gain? For a 130-pound person a five-pound increase would be noteworthy; whereas for a 210-pound individual a ten-pound weight gain would be noteworthy. Both would signal a call to action. Incidentally, for most people, over a lifetime, noteworthy weight shifts are all but inevitable. Nevertheless, you should **consider a noteworthy weight change a warning that you may be losing control of your weight and that you need to intervene to head off a potentially significant weight gain**.

If you need to lose five or ten pounds to get back to your best weight, go on a short-term mini diet. Revisit the Weight Loss Prediction tables and determine the calorie level needed to lose about two pounds per week. For example, a 40-year-old moderately active 130-pound female on a 1,200-Calorie diet, should be able to lose five pounds in approximately 18 days, and a 40-year-old moderately active 220-pound male should be able to lose ten pounds in approximately 24 days on a 1,800-Calorie diet.

Once back to your best weight, revisit and analyze your weight maintenance eating and exercise routines and make any adjustments needed to keep your weight on target. Furthermore, appreciate that in order to maintain a proper weight level you may have to go on a number of short-term mini diets over your lifetime to correct small weight maintenance calorie eating errors.

Keys to Life-Long Weight Control

As with most pursuits, the earlier in life you begin the better. But regardless of your age, the sooner you start a weight-control program the easier it will be and the more time you will have to reap the benefits. So start on the path to sure weight control now! Despite all the detailed information presented in this book the path to life-long weight control is actually deceptively simple, and can be reduced to five basic keys. Assuming you have had a medical checkup, the five basic keys to life-long weight control are:

Key 1: If you are in maintenance mode, know your maintenance calorie value, i.e., how many calories you can eat to neither gain nor lose weight. Periodically you might experience a noteworthy weight gain. If this happens immediately go on a mini-diet.

Key 2: Practice good nutrition by eating a variety of foods from each food group – all within your caloric allowance.

Key 3: Engage in moderate strength training at least two non-consecutive days per week.

Key 4: Engage in some form of moderate aerobic exercise every single day of the year. That is right every day!

LIFE-LONG FITNESS

There are lots of reasons to get fit: a longer life expectancy, less illness, a healthful appearance, the ability to work (and play) with vigor and an energy reserve for emergencies. To repeat what was said earlier, people who undertake a physical fitness program and attain a heightened level of fitness, report a dramatic reduction in chronic fatigue, an improved ability to relax, more energy for day-to-day tasks, firmer muscles and increased strength. In short, they feel better and look better too!

Why then is it so easy to become a dropout when fitness offers such wonderful health benefits? A fitness plan may be the missing link to getting and staying fit. Dr. Kanaar was a wonderful swimmer. (He.was the oldest person to swim around the island of Manhattan.) Dr. Kanaar not only taught me to be a more efficient swimmer, but at the same time he convinced me that it was especially **important for an individual starting a physical fitness program to set goals, have a plan and keep a fitness log.**

Everyone's personal goals and plan of attack will be different. Let us assume your goals are to lose 20 pounds and improve your overall health and fitness. First, commit yourself and start immediately. (Buy a notebook, or use your smart phone, because you will need to put your goals and plans in writing.) Next, plan how you are going to attain these goals. Broadly speaking, your overall plan might be to stop smoking; to begin a weight loss diet; and to start exercising. You must, however, be more specific and develop a detailed plan that indicates the when and how you are going to stop smoking, lose weight, etcetera. You might make up your mind to stop "cold turkey," or to enter a smoking secession program. Note the date you plan to start and the date you expect to be smoke free. Put it in writing!

For the weight loss portion of your plan, decide if you are going to go it alone or join some sort of clinical or non-clinical program.   [All the information you need for a do-it-yourself weight loss program is in this eBook.] If you settle on a do-it-yourself program, again note the diet calorie level, milestone dates for weight loss, etc. Put it in writing!

Then choose an exercise routine. Again using the principles covered in this book devise a realistic plan with time, place, type of exercise and frequency. Put it writing!

By now you must appreciate why you need a notebook. Once you actually start implementing your plan, you should also keep an exercise log and a food log to record your progress. An all-in-one fitness log that includes exercise as well as food is recommended. As you progress, periodically update your fitness plan. Enlist the support of your family and friends and do not forget to reward yourself when you reach a milestone – for a job well done!

The Keys to Total Fitness

As with most pursuits, the earlier in life you begin the better. But regardless of your age, the sooner you start a fitness program the easier it will be to get in shape and the more time you will have to reap the benefits. So for less illness, for a longer life expectancy, for a healthful appearance, start on the path to physical fitness now!

Despite all the detailed information presented in this book the path to life-long fitness is actually deceptively simple, and can be reduced to five basic keys. Assuming you have had a medical checkup, the five basic keys to life-long fitness are:

Key 1: Stop smoking and limit the consumption of alcoholic beverages. For some this will be difficult but both are absolutely necessary for life-long fitness.

Key 2: Keep your weight under control. Know your maintenance calorie value, i.e., how many calories you can eat to neither gain nor lose weight. Periodically you might experience a noteworthy weight gain. If this happens go on a mini-diet.

Key 3: Practice good nutrition by eating a variety of foods from each food group – all within your caloric allowance.

Key 4: Engage in moderate strength training at least two non-consecutive days a week.

Key 5: Engage in some form of moderate aerobic exercise every single day of the year. That is right every day! (If need be, cut back your aerobic workout on the days you do your strength exercises.)

To repeat, make every effort to engage in some form of moderate aerobic exercise every single day of the year! And try to exercise at the same time every day. This will probably mean rearranging priorities and putting exercise close to the top of your list. Soon exercise will become a part of your daily routine and you will not feel right unless you have had your daily run, or daily walk, etc.

Sure, there will be some days when it may seem impossible to fit exercise into your hectic schedule. Everyone would like to be able to workout for an uninterrupted hour, but the good news is that studies have shown that workouts as short as 15 minutes can improve your health. So on those very hectic, crazy days, try to fit in several 15-minute workouts whenever you can. Do the best with the time you have.

Any other occasional additional exercise such as a round of golf on the weekend, a game of handball, cross-country skiing, attending a yoga class, is fine, beneficial, but should be considered secondary to your daily aerobic workout.

Make It Happen

At this point, you have everything you need to succeed. You have an understanding of the fundamentals of exercise, nutrition and weight control. You have set realistic fitness goals, and you have a good fitness plan. If you combine all these with intense desire you'll be unstoppable. Your fitness regimen will work wonders and will have you looking and feeling better both physically and mentally. And when you look and feel your best, your spirit will soar. So as you start on the road to fitness, be aware that you are well prepared for success and always keep in mind how good you'll feel when you reach your goals.

Disclaimer

This book offers general meal planning, nutrition and weight control information. It is not a medical manual and the author does not claim to be medically qualified. The material in this book is not intended to be a substitute for medical counseling. Everyone should have a medical checkup before beginning a physical fitness program. Moreover, the physician conducting the medical exam should be made aware of and should approve the specific nutrition, exercise and weight control program planned. Additionally, while the author and publisher have made every effort to ensure the accuracy of the information in this book, they make no representations or warranties regarding its accuracy or completeness. Further, neither the author nor publisher assume liability for any medical problems that might result from applying the methods in this book, or for any loss of profit, or any other commercial damages, including but not limited to special, incidental, consequential or other damages, and any such liability is hereby expressly disclaimed.

www.ingramcontent.com/pod-product-compliance
Lightning Source LLC
Chambersburg PA
CBHW031127250726
48655CB00002B/552